2

THE

HOLLYWO☆D TRAINER™

WEIGHT-LOSS PLAN

Jeanette Jenkins

· · · ☆ · · ·

G. P. PUTNAM'S SONS

New York

THE

HOLLYWO☆D TRAINER™

WEIGHT-LOSS PLAN

21 DAYS

to Make Healthy Living

a Lifetime Habit

G. P. PUTNAM'S SONS
Publishers Since 1838
Published by the Penguin Group
Penguin Group (USA) Inc., 375 Hudson Street, New York, New York 10014, USA • Penguin Group (Canada),
90 Eglinton Avenue East, Suite 700, Toronto, Ontario M4P 2Y3, Canada (a division of Pearson Penguin Canada Inc.) •
Penguin Books Ltd, 80 Strand, London WC2R 0RL, England • Penguin Ireland, 25 St Stephen's Green, Dublin 2, Ireland
(a division of Penguin Books Ltd) • Penguin Group (Australia), 250 Camberwell Road, Camberwell, Victoria 3124, Australia
(a division of Pearson Australia Group Pty Ltd) • Penguin Books India Pvt Ltd, 11 Community Centre, Panchsheel Park,
New Delhi–110 017, India • Penguin Group (NZ), 67 Apollo Drive, Rosedale, North Shore 0745, Auckland, New Zealand (a division of
Pearson New Zealand Ltd) • Penguin Books (South Africa) (Pty) Ltd, 24 Sturdee Avenue, Rosebank, Johannesburg 2196, South Africa

Penguin Books Ltd, Registered Offices: 80 Strand, London WC2R 0RL, England

Library of Congress Cataloging-in-Publication Data

Jenkins, Jeanette.
The Hollywood trainer weight-loss plan : 21 days to make healthy living a lifetime habit / Jeanette Jenkins.
p.   cm.
Includes index.
ISBN 978-0-399-15374-7
1. Weight loss.   2. Nutrition.   3. Exercise.   4. Physical fitness.   5. Health.   I. Title.
RM222.2.J464   2007   2007001821
613.2'5—dc22

Printed in the United States of America
1   3   5   7   9   10   8   6   4   2

BOOK DESIGN BY MEIGHAN CAVANAUGH

Neither the publisher nor the author is engaged in rendering professional advice or services to the individual reader. The ideas, procedures, and suggestions contained in this book are not intended as a substitute for consulting with your physician. All matters regarding your health require medical supervision. Neither the author nor the publisher shall be liable or responsible for any loss or damage allegedly arising from any information or suggestion in this book.

The recipes contained in this book are to be followed exactly as written. The publisher is not responsible for your specific health or allergy needs that may require medical supervision. The publisher is not responsible for any adverse reactions to the recipes contained in this book.

While the author has made every effort to provide accurate telephone numbers and Internet addresses at the time of publication, neither the publisher nor the author assumes any responsibility for errors, or for changes that occur after publication. Further, the publisher does not have any control over and does not assume any responsibility for author or third-party websites or their content.

HOLLYWO☆D TRAINER is a trademark of The Hollywood Trainer, Inc.

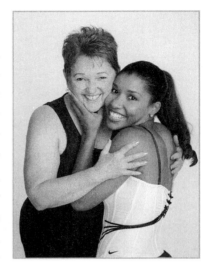

I grew up in public housing with my mother, Karen Jones, older brother, Roger Jenkins, and older sister, Camille Jenkins. Throughout my childhood and adolescence my mother gave 99 percent of her time to her children and, like so many parents who put their family's needs above their own, she simply didn't take care of her own health. In March 2006, my mother was rushed to the emergency room of her local hospital with a gallbladder attack. While I knew this wasn't an immediately life-threatening episode, I felt the pain of what it would be like to deal with my mother's passing. After she recovered, I moved her to Los Angeles to be near me but, equally important, I knew for sure that there was no way I could work as a fitness expert and not use my expertise to motivate and change my mother's life. I took her on as a regular client. At age sixty she has been able to change her life! Since her illness she's lost weight (gone down three dress sizes), lowered her cholesterol, strengthened her heart, improved her cardiovascular fitness, balance, and stability, and most important, she is looking and feeling great!

My goal in writing this book is to give a workable plan with all the information, advice, and encouragement needed to change anyone's life. I hope and pray that this book will help those who are suffering from preventable diseases. My mother was able to do it, and so can you!

I dedicate this book to my mother and to all parents who sacrifice so much for their children. Thank you, Mom, for showing me the valuable gift of giving because it has added so much happiness to my life!

—*Jeanette*

CONTENTS

Part Five

YOU HAVE TO MOVE IT TO LOSE IT!

Part Six

HEALTHY HABITS FOR LIFE

FOREWORD

When Jeanette told me she was writing a book, I said, "Gee, that's swell!" No. Just kidding—I never say swell. But I did agree to write this foreword because I believe that she has some lifesaving advice to give to everyone. I am a witness to the writing of this book, but more important, I have enjoyed the countless benefits of what Jeanette has put into it. This book will be a blessing to your life, just as Jeanette has been to mine.

Jeanette is absolutely the most knowledgeable trainer I have ever worked with. She has this wonderful energy and a great spirit, which she brings to every training session, shares with everyone around her every day, and has put into the pages of this book. With Jeanette's program, I saw amazing results in a short time. I lost twenty-five pounds in less than six weeks—and I did it the natural way, by eating right and exercising smart. And, for once in my life, I just listened and did what was asked of me. We worked out a program that I was able to follow, and she showed me not only *what* to do but *why* I was doing it. Because she knows so much about what it takes to get fit, I was able to reach my goals—and surpass them—by putting my time and energy into eating properly and exercising efficiently. Most important, she helped me find the motivation to stay with the program—and make a lifetime commitment to good health.

But losing the weight and getting in shape are only part of the story. Jeanette's program is not *just* about getting the pounds off and looking good. Because Jeanette's passion is about getting people healthy in *every* way—mentally, spiritually, and physically—she is unlike any other trainer that I've worked with. Most of them focus only on the look: the six-pack abs or the tight booty. In other words, they promise to give you a movie star's body, which is just not realistic for most of us, including me. And I *am* a movie star!

Over the years I've been impressed not only by Jeanette's deep knowledge about health and fitness, but also by her effort to push herself to learn more. She's never satisfied with the way things are, especially if she thinks they can be better. It seems that every day there's some new diet or exercise fad—and lots of people promising the magic bullet or an instant weight-loss scheme. It's sometimes hard to sort them all out. That's where Jeanette comes in. She tries to make us more aware of how to be healthy and how to take care of ourselves, not by judging us but by teaching us healthier alternatives and how to incorporate them realistically into our daily living. She's not only done her homework, but she's also put it all together in a way that anyone can understand and follow, and, like me, can see and feel real change in just twenty-one days.

I used to smoke—yes, I know, it's a nasty habit—but I was able to quit with the help of a book called *Freshstart: 21 Days to Stop Smoking.* (The book is out of print, but you might still be able to find a used copy online.) The book and my own experience convinced me that it does take twenty-one days to kick a habit. (I don't know about the science behind this theory but you'll be able to try it for yourself.) Jeanette has taken this idea one step further: if you can *break* a bad habit in twenty-one days, then you can certainly *create* a good habit in the same amount of time. But I can't forget to give Jeanette credit for helping me to quit by being a positive influence in my life so that when I was ready to do it, I had someone to support me. (Creating a support system is one of the key principles of Jeanette's program, no matter what goal you are trying to accomplish.) Healthy living can become a habit for a lifetime. This is the promise of this book, and it's a promise that you can rely on if you are willing to take the necessary steps. Remember, it's not just about *reading* this book, it's about doing what you know is right and looking to Jeanette for the best way to do it.

With Jeanette's guidance, I've changed the way I live, especially when it comes to eating. I eat a lot more organic foods (and you'll learn more about this in the book) and I've taken to heart her advice about portion control. She gives lots of cool little tricks about how to burn fat even longer by avoiding certain foods and sugary drinks after a workout. The recipes, menus, and nutritional information that she provides really helped me to take control of my eating.

In terms of working out, I have never met anyone who knew so many different moves. There's no way you'll ever get bored. I've always known that there is a general way to get fit, but Jeanette has shown me so many specifics that have made a tremendous difference. If there is a particular area of my body that I want to strengthen—like my knees or shoulders, to help me do more physical things for my job—she knows ways to help build up those particular muscles. But she also knows working other muscles is essential because our bodies are not made of isolated muscles and bones. Jeanette's a real know-it-all in the best sense of the word! She knows. She knows, okay!

But here's the real deal: Jeanette knows how to keep me motivated, and how I can motivate myself when she's not around. Remember the idea of creating a good habit in twenty-one days? There was a time when the thought of exercise would just make me think: forget about it. Now I *have* to exercise. Even if I'm feeling lazy, my body just craves it. Whether it's bike riding outside, walking home from a restaurant instead of driving, or doing a few crunches before bed, exercise has become a habit! (And another thing I learned from Miss-Know-It-All is that I don't just have to be in a gym, because there are a lot of ways to exercise that don't involve fancy equipment.)

For me, life is for the living. I am not the kind of person who's always going to listen to every so-called expert. I'm a little too strong-headed for that. But I have enough sense to want to be around to keep doing the things I like to do, whether it's jumping off cliffs in Jamaica, hiking mountains in Hawaii, eating really good food in Italy or Paris, or just walking through some museum. I know that the healthier I am the more I can appreciate what I've got, and what I've got to look forward to.

I just encourage everyone to get off their lazy butts and hit it, baby! I think the Hollywood Trainer Weight-Loss Plan is a great way to jump off a new life!

—*Queen Latifah*

Part One

THE 7 SIMPLE STEPS TO

HEALTHIER LIVING

The Hollywood Trainer Weight-Loss Plan is based on seven simple steps that are easy to discuss but a little more challenging to implement in everyday life. The problem is one of balance, which you must have in order to live a healthy life and fulfill goals. How do you manage your time effectively so you can get things done stress-free and enjoy the journey? Many successful and happy people agree on a few things: create a plan, don't sweat the small stuff, be prepared, follow and believe in your faith, do what is in your heart, and live your life. Again, these tips are easy to talk about but much harder to follow.

In more than seventeen years of teaching and training thousands of clients I have observed a few patterns in individuals who are mentally, physically, and spiritually healthy. The common thread: seven simple steps to healthy living that will be thoroughly outlined in this section. I have incorporated them into a comprehensive step-by-step holistic twenty-one-day plan to help you create a lifestyle that will decrease your stress and anxiety levels, prepare your daily meals and workouts, and live your best life.

1

IT'S TIME TO CHANGE YOUR LIFE

Why are some people able to succeed in adopting new healthy habits while others are not? Be honest: do you have weights or exercise equipment at home that go unused? Do you pay for a gym membership that you never use? Do you read books and articles and know exactly what you need to do, but just don't get around to doing it? Do you know friends or loved ones who have suffered from diseases that could have been prevented by better nutrition or more exercise, but *still* haven't learned to make the changes to your lifestyle that you *know* you need to make? Why are so many of us out of touch with our health and ourselves? What exactly is the problem?

The problem is that as we speed through our lives, working hard at jobs and taking care of families, we are not taking the time we need to connect our minds, hearts, and souls to the physical conditions of our bodies. So what's the solution? The Hollywood Trainer Weight-Loss Plan will give you all the tools you need to help you finally make that necessary and life-changing connection. Now, I know your next question: how is this program going to be any different from all of the other diets and workouts you've tried in the past? Keep reading, because there are several elements that separate this program from others. I have taken the most important elements from my seventeen years of training, elements that have helped thousands of my students, clients, and colleagues become successful, to create a twenty-one-day holistic program that works so well I put my own mother on it! So read on and you will be convinced that this twenty-one-day program is different from anything else you have tried!

IT TAKES ONLY 21 DAYS TO CHANGE YOUR LIFE

The Hollywood Trainer Weight-Loss Plan outlines a twenty-one-day strategy for programming new behaviors that you will ultimately adopt for life. Experts agree and research shows that a habit is formed after just twenty-one days of consistent action. My plan will teach you to integrate new, healthy behaviors into your day-to-day life over three weeks, at the end of which these "new behaviors" will be a lifestyle.

FORGE THE VITAL CONNECTION
BETWEEN THE MIND AND THE BODY

Part of the reason so many Americans are overweight in the first place is that we are not taking the time to connect our minds, hearts, and souls to our physical bodies. Taking time each day to be still and acknowledge where you are and what you've been through is imperative to reclaiming your body's natural equilibrium. Every day of this program contains exercises to help you find this balance, which in turn will help you succeed in changing your lifestyle for good. Any weight-loss program that disregards the mental and spiritual aspects of physical health is not addressing the full problem, and cannot help you make the complete transformation to better health for life.

SEE AND FEEL THE RESULTS

Most people are going to give up on a new program if they don't see immediate results. There are numerous benefits to working out, but if your number one goal is to lose weight and burn off body fat, you're going to lose steam if you don't see that happening. On my program, you are required to take your measurements every week, so you will actually measure the results on paper as well as see them on your body. (The many before-and-after photos and testimonials that appear throughout this book and on my Web site, www.thehollywoodtrainer.com, provide additional motivation if you start to lose heart.) Knowing that you are moving toward your goal will steel you against quitting, and will keep your eyes on the prize—a healthier, happier you.

LEARN ABOUT YOUR BODY

It's a fact: people who understand their bodies and how they work are more likely to succeed at any fitness program. Haven't you always wanted to know exactly how your body burns calories and fat? Aren't you more likely not to skip breakfast, and not to load up on complex carbs in the evening, if you know the reasons why you shouldn't? Wouldn't you like to understand why circuit training is better and more effective than straight cardio and weights? This book gives you the answers you want in a simple, friendly format so that the knowledge will stay with you for a lifetime.

YOU CAN DO IT

I see it happen all the time—people buy DVDs or books, or join classes, only to discover that the exercises are too advanced for their level of fitness. This leads to discouragement and quitting, which chips away at people's self-confidence and self-esteem, until they think that they will never be able to get into shape. Well, they're wrong. With the Hollywood Trainer Weight-Loss Plan, that problem has been eliminated. When selecting the exercises for this program, I considered each one and made sure that any beginner, regardless of fitness level or weight problem, would be able to execute each movement. It's time to ditch your fears and insecurities—this is the program for you.

NO MORE EXCUSES

We all know that time is one of our most valuable commodities; in fact, one of the excuses people use *not* to start working out is that they just don't have the time. Well, if it takes you thirty to forty-five minutes to get to the gym, forty-five to sixty minutes to complete your workout, twenty minutes to shower and change, then thirty to forty-five minutes to get back home or to work, then no wonder you don't have time! Most of us don't have three hours a day to devote to working out. That's why my program can be done either at the gym, or entirely in the comfort of your own home. Working out at the gym surrounded by other people can give you great energy—but it's important to find a gym that is close or easy to get to during off-peak traffic hours. If you don't have a gym close by, or on days when you are in a rush, you can work my program as soon as you roll out of bed without having to worry about what you're wearing or what you look like. So, no more excuses! My program is so convenient you can't help but succeed.

MOTIVATE AND INSPIRE YOURSELF

We all dance to our own beat, finding motivation and inspiration in different places. Of course we all hope to be able to turn to others when we need help getting through a rough patch, but there are times when our friends and loved ones are just not available. Therefore, it's crucial that you find your own tangible sources of inspiration that are always available at a moment's notice. My program teaches you how to identify what motivates *you* so that you can be your own best support system on the road to a healthy life.

HOW—AND WHY—TO BUILD A SUPPORT SYSTEM

It takes a village to do many things, including changing your life. Without the support of people around you, it is much harder as you embark on your journey to a happier, healthier you. I'm going to show you how to get the help you need. Let's face it, there are going to be days when you may be at the mercy of stressful or emotional circumstances, and, like anyone, you may need a little encouragement to stay on track. Any program that ignores the importance of building a supportive environment leaves a gaping hole for people to fall through to failure. After all, if it were easy to make these lifestyle changes, everyone would be doing it all the time, and obesity rates in this country wouldn't be so high.

CREATE HEALTHY HABITS THAT LAST A LIFETIME

This program brings benefits that you will reap for the rest of your life. The initial twenty-one-day commitment is the window of time when your learning curve will be the steepest, and when you will be going through the most dramatic changes. But the habits that you learn and adopt over the three-week course of my program will also put you on track for a lifetime of health and happiness, and added longevity.

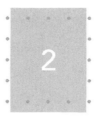

THE 7 SIMPLE STEPS TO SUCCESS

The Hollywood Trainer Weight-Loss Plan provides a holistic program that will teach you how to get and stay healthy. Unlike many fitness books and programs, this one is designed with *you* in mind, and I have made allowances for the fact that you will be coming to this with your own unique needs and goals; this book is structured so that you can jump in at any level and grow with me.

I take every personal client through a series of tests to make a full assessment of her level of physical readiness and mental commitment. I also take detailed measurements to record against future progress. I consider this to be an essential first step for any fitness program because you have to know your starting point in order to fully understand how to reach your goals. In addition, the more accurately you can track your progress, the more motivated you will be to stay the course. Before you start my program, you should undergo this same thorough assessment, using the forms, questionnaires, instructions, and charts you will find in Part 2, Getting to Know Your Mind, Body, and Spirit. Once you have a realistic notion of where you're starting from, I will help you set and achieve your personal goals.

7 STEPS TO SUCCESS

At the core of my program are seven simple steps to healthy living that will guarantee improved health and weight loss. In the course of helping thousands of people lose weight and change their lives, I've learned that these steps are the key to success.

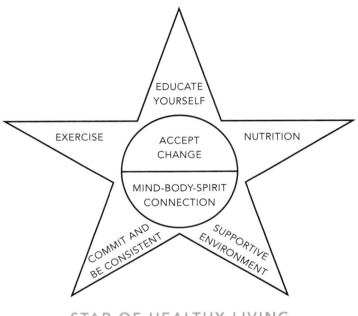

STAR OF HEALTHY LIVING

For this program, I have incorporated these seven steps into the twenty-one-day program. Follow all of them and you will achieve your goals just like the thousands of clients I have helped over the years.

1. ACCEPT CHANGE

Whether you're a hundred pounds overweight or just a little out of shape, it's important to accept the fact that the choices you've made have brought you to where you are. Once you take responsibility for your present condition, and understand that you are not a victim of your past, you claim the power to shape your future. No matter what may have held you back from succeeding up to now, you still have the power to change the choices you make. I've had clients come to me with all kinds of problems they thought were insurmountable: late-night snacking, excessive alcohol consumption, depression, emotional eating, fatigue, sugar and bread addiction—you name it, I've heard it and helped people get over it. (Many of their testimonials appear throughout the book.) If you want a different outcome then you have to accept that what you have been doing up until now is not working, so you must make a change. Remember, only you have the power to change, but I will help you discover it.

2. MAKE THE MIND-BODY-SPIRIT CONNECTION

Perhaps the most vital step to any lasting lifestyle change is to understand that you have to love yourself enough to want to take care of yourself. You need to learn how to acknowledge your physical body in its present moment. Over the next three weeks you will be doing exercises in meditation and spiritual affirmation—every new day will begin with a reconfirmation of the qualities you possess that you love, and all the many reasons you owe it to yourself to take care of your health before tending to everyone else in your life.

3. EXERCISE: YOU HAVE TO MOVE IT TO LOSE IT!

We first appeared on this earth as hunters and gatherers, with bodies designed to move accordingly. In today's world of efficient conveniences, the reality is that we have to go out of our way to burn calories. Okay, so working out isn't your favorite thing in the world. You can burn an additional 300 to 500 calories a day just by making small changes. If you educate yourself and structure it right, working out can be fun; and the progress you will start to see right away will be a powerful motivation to stay the course. One of the goals of this program is to help you find ways of making exercising enjoyable and all about you, so that you are able to incorporate it into your life for good, and start reaping those amazing benefits.

4. NUTRITION: YOU ARE WHAT YOU EAT

When it comes to nutrition, it's easy to put health on the back burner for the sake of convenience. But we also have to understand that what we eat every day has a direct effect on our health and well-being. Most of us can recite the words to dozens of our favorite songs, but we have little notion of what's in the food we eat. When was the last time you read a food label? Most of us stopped when food ingredients became unpronounceable chemical compounds, especially in packaged diet foods. Along with a comprehensive section on the nutritional information you need to make the right choices, each day of the program includes a full daily meal plan with quick and delicious recipes to help you kick-start your new, healthy lifestyle.

5. EDUCATE YOURSELF

In order to achieve lasting results, it's crucial that you acquire a basic understanding of how your physical and mental acts affect your body and your overall well-being. Aside from what you will learn about nutrition and exercise in the respective parts of this book, each day of the program features an important lesson about the science of weight loss and fat burning, which will provide a focus for your day's activities and reinforce the goals you've set for yourself. Knowledge of spirit, nutrition, and exercise can be converted to weight loss, longevity, and quality of life.

6. COMMIT AND BE CONSISTENT

We are what we repeatedly do. Excellence, therefore, is not an act, but a habit.
—*Aristotle*

When one of my clients, Kimberly Brant from the BET Foundation's Healthy BET Fitness Challenge, put this Aristotle quote on her daily journal e-mails, it made me realize that the defining difference between those who are successful at losing weight and those who can't seem to budge the scale is *consistency* once they have made the commitment.

As you embark upon this life-changing process, it's crucial that you understand at every point along the way exactly where you are in your journey, and how you are going to get to the next level. Over the course of your work you will create valuable tools for journaling, planning, measuring, and logging your progress. Once you can gauge how well you're doing—mentally and physically—it will be that much easier to keep going.

7. CREATE A SUPPORTIVE ENVIRONMENT

Your chances of success are higher—and you'll have more fun—if you create a network of support. Whether it's a workout buddy, a family member to help cook a healthy meal, a mentor, or simply your faith, discover what motivates and inspires you. And throughout this book you will find an array of innovative methods that you can adopt or adapt for making your surroundings much more conducive to your ultimate success.

You can experience true transformation only when you take a holistic approach to your health. By absorbing all of the seven simple steps to healthy living on a regular basis, you leave no room for failure. The magic of my program is the sum of its parts—so skipping even one step is not an option.

Are you ready to take these first steps toward a healthier, happier life? You know you want to—I'm telling you that you can. Let's get started!

GETTING THE MOST OUT OF THE HOLLYWOOD TRAINER WEIGHT-LOSS PLAN

Before you begin, you should take a moment to read—and follow—these important tips. Like reading the full list of ingredients before you start to make a recipe, it is critical to know what you'll need to make the plan work best for you.

This book is full of information, but there will be specific pieces that will create an *aha!* moment for you, and those are the things that you will want to put into your personal journal. Over the course of the twenty-one days, I encourage you to fill your journal with facts, quotes, recipes, or whatever bits of information will help you achieve your goal. This journal will grow with you, and you can add to it from other resources as well.

1. Make your personal Hollywood Trainer Weight-Loss journal using a three-ring binder with dividers to create the following sections: Mental/Physical/Spiritual, Measurements, Nutrition, Exercise, and Education. You will also need five clear plastic binder pockets, one for each section of your journal, to hold newspaper articles, notes from friends, photos, or whatever you'll collect as you work your way through the program. In many cases you will be using the pre-designed forms provided in this book or at my Web site, but you will also want to include some lined sheets to write your own entries. (Many people may want to create e-journals, which you can also do by downloading all the forms from www.thehollywoodtrainer.com.)

2. Make photocopies from this book or download and print the forms, and put them in the appropriate sections of your journal, as designated. (Forms 1 through 6 are found in Part 2: Getting to Know Your Mind, Body, and Spirit; forms 7 through 11 can be found in the Appendix.)

Form 1: Connecting Mind, Body, and Spirit (Mental/Physical/Spiritual)
Form 2: Personal Contract for a New, Healthy Life (Mental/Physical/Spiritual)
Form 3: Pre-Exercise Health Screen (Measurements)
Form 4: Body Composition Assessment (Measurements)
Form 5: Daily Calorie Intake and Output Charts (Measurements)

Form 6: Your Personal Fitness Profile (Measurements)

Form 7: Daily Food Log (Nutrition)

Form 8: Cardiorespiratory Training Log (Exercise)

Form 9: Circuit Training Log (Exercise)

Form 10: Flexibility Training Log (Exercise)

Form 11: Before-and-After Photos

3. Make an appointment with your doctor or other health-care professional. I recommend that you get a full physical. Take your journal and your book and let your doctor know that you plan on starting a new fitness regimen. Find out if there are any specific restrictions or guidelines that you must follow based on your current health condition. Ask your doctor to fill in your measurements for blood pressure and cholesterol levels on Form 3. Some doctors may also be able to conduct a cardiorespiratory test or stress test, which is a more accurate variation of the aerobic test provided in the fitness assessment.

4. Schedule a 60-minute appointment with yourself—or with a certified trainer—to go through the Body Composition Assessment (Form 4) and Daily Calorie Intake and Output Charts (Form 5).

5. Schedule a 60-minute time slot in which you will complete the fitness tests I've provided in Part 2 (Form 6). You may also wish to complete these tests with a certified personal trainer, but it is not necessary.

6. Get out your daily planner and schedule your workouts for the next three weeks. That's right! You have to find time to fit in a 30- to 60-minute workout six days a week for the next twenty-one days. I find that the best time for a workout is first thing in the morning—it boosts energy levels and you start your day by taking the time to do something good for yourself. Also, it's out of the way and you don't have to worry about trying to fit a workout into your day once things get hectic. Having said that, it's hard for many of us to devote the early morning to ourselves, and any time that you can commit to is time that you can make count.

7. Review the daily meal plans and recipes for the first seven days provided in Part 3: 21 Days That Will Change Your Life, and Part 4: Eating for Life, making any substitutions according to allergies or budget.

Part Two

GETTING TO KNOW YOUR MIND, BODY, AND SPIRIT

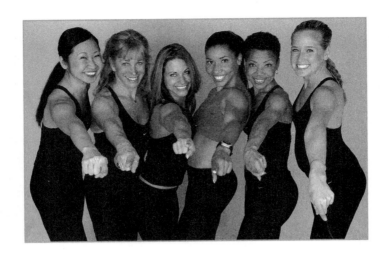

This part of the book is dedicated to helping you fine-tune and tailor the twenty-one-day plan to meet your needs, because there is no such thing as one size fits all. I have provided questionnaires and self-tests that you'll need to measure and record your own mental and physical strengths and weaknesses. I like to compare this process to creating a personal budget. To get your finances in order you have to take a look at your income, spending habits, savings, debt, ongoing financial obligations, and goals. To do the same for your health, you need to look at your physical, mental, and emotional state—from cardiovascular functions to muscular strength, from stress levels to personal issues. Using the tools provided here, you have a starting point so you can chart your progress with several measurements instead of focusing only on what the scale says.

Getting to know yourself—your past experiences and your current habits—is the most valuable part of training. There is no way I can help you achieve your goals until you put all of your cards on the table. The more you know, the more you will get out of this program. Once you understand and take note of your strengths and challenges, then it will be much easier to make positive changes. Besides, getting to know your *self* is also a lot of fun and it will motivate you to get *results*. You will be surprised by all the things you discover about *yourself*! Get started—it is time to learn a few new things about *you*!

THE STARTING POINT
ON THE ROAD TO SUCCESS

You are about to turn your life around. But before you can do that with any hope of success, you have to take a long hard look at where you are right now. Are you happy with the way you feel? With the way you look? Do you wake up and embrace the day or wish you could hide from it? These are just some of the questions you need to ask yourself before you can really take control of your life and your future. It is time to measure your success by focusing on your own individual starting point, progress, and attainable goals. Too often, men and women compare themselves to social standards of health and beauty that are plastered across magazine covers and television screens. Others measure their success by standards placed on them by their parents, friends, partners, bosses, jobs, or community. Well, this program is not about any of them, it's about you. It is time to start measuring your progress by focusing on yourself, your starting point, your goals, your progress, and your successes.

When I take on a new client, the first few sessions are all about getting to know them: where they are now, where they want to be, what's holding them back, and how they can overcome their obstacles and achieve success. To get a full and accurate assessment of a new client's current situation, I put each client through a series of tests, ask them a lot of questions, and take extensive body measurements; all of this information is then recorded so that the client has a detailed account of where they're starting from. Not only does this provide a multidimensional point of reference as they start to transform their health and their body, but it also serves as a better indicator of their overall health and fitness than just getting on the scale or looking in the mirror. Health comes from the inside out, not the other way around. If you're really committed to health for life, losing weight is only part of the picture. Your body is made up of 60 to 70 percent water and 30 to 40 percent muscle (lean body tissue), connective tissues (bones, ligaments, tendons), and internal organs and fat (adipose tissue). According to the American Council on Exercise and the American Council of Sports Medicine, an obese female has 32 percent or more of her body weight composed of fat, and an obese male 25 percent or more of his body weight composed of fat. When you lose weight, you need to be sure that you are not just losing water and muscle, but that you are actually decreasing body fat and improving your blood pressure, cholesterol levels, mental health, cardiovascular health, bone density, muscular strength, muscular endurance, and flexibility. These are the things that really matter to your health, and by monitoring them from the very beginning, you can improve these numbers, decreasing your risk of numerous health-related diseases such as hypertension, diabetes, heart attack, stroke, cancer, osteoporosis, and hardening of the arteries, to name just a few.

So now it's your turn to own up and get honest about the shape you're in. What follows are the same tests I use for all my clients. Getting to know yourself is an exciting part of this process, so grab a pencil and get started.

4

MAKING THE MIND-BODY-SPIRIT CONNECTION

You probably spend a lot of time running around tending to others or exerting yourself at work. It's time to slow down and be present in this moment. Caring for others and working hard are important and wonderful things to do, but don't forget to take care of yourself. This first questionnaire will help you consider yourself and your feelings so that you can begin to draw yourself away from the sidelines of your own life and jump into the driver's seat.

Take the time to reflect on the different ways you feel about yourself in different situations and environments. If your feelings about yourself change depending on the circumstances, ask yourself why. Remember, even though your environment changes, *you are still the same wonderful person.*

You don't have to allow anyone else's standards of beauty to define you. You must define yourself so that you have a positive way of standing firm against the negative stereotypes and small-mindedness of others that may have eroded your self-confidence in the past.

Photocopy the following pages or download Form 1: Connecting Mind, Body, and Spirit from www.thehollywoodtrainer.com. Answer all of the questions as thoughtfully and honestly as you can, and then put the completed form in the Mental/Physical/Spiritual section of your journal.

CONNECTING MIND, BODY, AND SPIRIT

1. How do you feel about yourself right now?

2. How do you feel about yourself when you are at work?

3. How do you feel about yourself when you are with your family?

4. How do you feel about yourself when you are with your friends?

5. How do you feel about yourself when you are going out to social events and meeting new people?

6. What are the qualities that define you as a person? In all of the various environments you move through in life—work, social events, parenting, being a partner, being a friend—what are the consistent character traits and values that best describe you? (Be honest if you think that some of these traits may be less than positive. Don't judge yourself. In order to change, you have to recognize the things that need to be changed. And remember, only you will be reading this journal.)

7. Why have you been unsuccessful at losing weight, or keeping it off, in the past?

8. What do you think are your two unhealthiest habits?

9. What other unhealthy habits do you have that may not be associated with your weight?

10. Are you prepared to break these unhealthy habits and replace them with new, healthy ones?

11. What are your specific goals in the short term (three to twelve weeks)?

12. What are your specific goals in the mid term (six to twelve months) and long term (two years)?

Form 1: Connecting Mind, Body, and Spirit

SIGN ON THE DOTTED LINE

I want you to sign a contract between you and your health. Your body has had enough. It's tired of the junk food you eat on the fly, of not getting enough exercise, of being treated like your last priority. Now it's time for you to take responsibility so that you can change in the future.

Each of us has our own special challenges, whether it's getting up on time or cooking our own meals or taking time for prayer or reflection. This contract is the place to write down those things that you want to change because the plan that you are now following is not just a diet and exercise regimen, it is a new way of living.

An effective contract clearly outlines the responsibilities of all concerned parties, and the Personal Contract for a New, Healthy Life is no different. Photocopy or download Form 2: Personal Contract for a New, Healthy Life from www.thehollywoodtrainer.com. Place the completed and signed contract form in the Mental/Physical/Spiritual section of your journal as a reminder of your commitment to yourself. If you breach the contract, the only person you hurt is yourself.

PERSONAL CONTRACT FOR A NEW, HEALTHY LIFE

My personal short-term goals (three to twelve weeks) are:

1. _____
   _____

2. _____
   _____

3. _____
   _____

My personal mid- and long-term goals (six months to two years) are:

1. _____
   _____

2. _____
   _____

3. _____
   _____

I believe that I have the strength, power, desire, and commitment to break the following unhealthy habits:

1. _____
   _____
2. _____
   _____
3. _____
   _____

I am committing to form new, healthy habits by completing each and every step in the Hollywood Trainer Weight-Loss Plan so that I can reap the benefits of a healthy mind, body, and soul. At the end of the twenty-one days, I am going to take the valuable information I have learned and create my own personal program to continue my new, healthy life. I love myself and know that without my health I will be unable to help friends, family, and loved ones. I will make time for myself in order to be a stronger person for myself and others. I know that when my mind, body, and soul are healthy, I am able to give back to the universe.

I will commit to the following specific endeavors that have been difficult for me in the past.

1. _____
   _____
2. _____
   _____
3. _____
   _____

_____   _____
Signature   Date

Form 2: Personal Contract for a New, Healthy Life

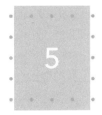

5

PRE-EXERCISE HEALTH SCREEN

You can perform most of the tests and questionnaires in this book in the privacy of your own home. But it's important to know your blood pressure and cholesterol levels, which you should get from your doctor or health-care provider before starting the exercise part of the program. Be sure to have the same person measure your levels each time you go for a follow-up. Make sure you inform your doctor about your new fitness regimen and ask if there are any specific guidelines that you need to follow based on your current state of health. Once you get your numbers, you will be all the more gratified to watch them improve. Photocopy or download Form 3: Pre-Exercise Health Screen, and put the completed form in the Measurements section of your journal.

PRE-EXERCISE HEALTH SCREEN

Today's date and time: _____

Who is taking your blood pressure and conducting the cholesterol test?

_____

	Today	*at 6 weeks*	*at 12 weeks*	*at 6 months*	*at 1 year*	*at 2 years*
RESTING HEART RATE						
BLOOD PRESSURE						
CHOLESTEROL LDL: HDL: TOTAL:						
TRIGLYCERIDES						

Doctor or health-care professional's recommendations:

_____

_____

_____

_____

Form 3: Pre-Exercise Health Screen

RESTING HEART RATE

You can take this measurement yourself. Resting heart rate must be taken first thing in the morning while you're still lying in bed, just after you've woken up. Place your index and middle fingers on your radial artery (the pulse point on your forearm close to your wrist) and count the number of beats in 60 seconds. There are no definitive standards for resting-heart-rate

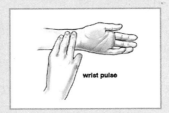

wrist pulse

classification, but on average the heart beats 60 to 80 times per minute when the body is at rest, and is generally lower in those who are physically fit. You may find that your resting heart rate will decrease as you start working out and your heart gets stronger. The heart is a muscle, and the stronger it becomes the more blood it can pump in one beat, thus requiring fewer beats per minute to circulate the blood through your body. As your arteries become less clogged and your body fat decreases, your heart will also be able to pump your blood through your body much more easily.

BLOOD PRESSURE AND CHOLESTEROL LEVELS

A doctor or health-care professional should take your blood pressure and draw some blood for a cholesterol test. Ask your health-care professional to spend five minutes with you to interpret your results, and ask if he or she has any recommendations for you as you start an exercise program or diet.

IDEAL LEVELS:
Blood pressure: less than 120/80 mm Hg (It's the top number that counts.)

Cholesterol:
    LDL (bad) cholesterol: below 100 mg/dl
    HDL (good) cholesterol: above 40 mg/dl
    Total cholesterol: below 200 mg/dl

Triglycerides: below 150 mg/dl

(All target levels are according to the American Heart Association.)

BODY COMPOSITION

Nothing's better than hopping on the scale and seeing that number drop. Unfortunately, when it comes to measuring your real health, the scale doesn't tell us much. Body weight is made up of fat, muscle, water, internal organs, bones, and connective tissues, so for a meaningful evaluation of your health, you need to know more about your body.

First, a few explanations of the various measures used and how to calculate them:

BODY MASS INDEX

Body mass index (BMI) is a measure of your weight relative to your height. To determine your BMI, use the equation below, provided by the Centers for Disease Control. Evidence has shown that an elevated BMI increases your risk of cancer, diabetes, hypertension, hypercholesterolemia, heart disease, and atherosclerosis. And yet results from the National Health and Nutrition Examination Survey indicate that more than 66 percent of the U.S. population is overweight or obese, and is consequently at risk of premature death.

$$\text{BMI} = \left(\frac{\text{Weight in Pounds}}{(\text{Height in Inches}) \times (\text{Height in Inches})} \right) \times 703$$

Now check your results against the standard as listed in the table below:

BMI	Weight Status
Below 18.5	Underweight
18.5–24.9	Normal
25.0–29.9	Overweight
30.0 and above	Obese

BODY FAT ANALYSIS

According to the American Council of Sports Medicine, body fat of more than 32 percent in women, or 25 percent in men, indicates increased risk for disease. There are currently several methods of measuring body fat. Here are the five most widely used: bioelectrical impedance, hydrostatic weighing, Bod Pod, body scan, and calipers. For the sake of accuracy, use two of the following four methods to measure your body fat, and when you retest make sure that you use the same two methods each time. Most body fat analysis is done by a personal trainer or health specialist, although some home devices are available.

BIOELECTRICAL IMPEDANCE

Bioelectrical impedance body fat analysis is based on the theory that fat is a poor electrical conductor containing little water (14 to 22 percent), and therefore impedes electrical current, while lean tissue is a good electrical conductor containing mostly water (90 percent) and electrolytes. In a bioelectrical impedance test, your total body water is measured and calculations of your body fat percentage are made, using basic assumptions about your hydration levels. You can get scales that measure body fat using the bioelectrical impedance method. The handheld Omron body fat monitor and foot pad scales by Tanita, Taylor, Soehnle, and Omron are available on Amazon.com and at Target, Wal-Mart, and Sports Authority. (More advanced methods of bioelectrical impedance analysis are also available at many gyms, doctors' offices, and health centers.) For the most accurate results, measure first thing in the morning or four hours after you last ate or drank; avoid alcohol consumption within forty-eight hours of testing; do not take diuretics within seven days of testing; and refrain from exercise for twelve hours before testing.

HYDROSTATIC WEIGHING ("DUNK TANK")

Hydrostatic weighing to determine body fat percentages is based on the assumption that density and specific gravity of lean tissue are greater than those of fat tissue. Thus, lean tissue will sink in water, and fat tissue will float. By comparing a test subject's mass measured underwater and out of the water, body fat percentage may be calculated using mathematical prediction. Hydrostatic weighing methodology assumes that the density of bone in humans is constant. Thus, differences in bone density will create test errors. African-Americans and trained athletes are now known to have a higher bone density than nonathletes and Caucasians. The elderly and Asians have considerably lower bone density. Specialized equations have been developed for use with African-American populations.

BOD POD

The Bod Pod was developed with grant funding from the National Institutes of Health and uses patented air-displacement technology. The Bod Pod technology is based on the same whole-body measurement principle as hydrostatic weighing (the "dunk tank") with one change. The Bod Pod displaces air instead of water so you don't have to get wet.

BODY SCAN

Body scan (or DEXA Scan) is currently the most widely used method to measure bone mineral density, but this device can also be used to measure body fat percentage and locate the parts of your body that carry the most fat. DEXA systems use a source that generates X-rays at two energies that can estimate three body compartments consisting of fat mass, lean body mass, and bone mass. DEXA also has the ability to determine body composition in defined regions, such as the arms, legs, and trunk. DEXA measurements are based in part on the assumption that the hydration of fat-free mass remains constant at 73 percent. Hydration, however, can vary from 67 to 85 percent, and can be variable in certain disease states. Other assumptions used to derive body composition estimates are considered proprietary by DEXA manufacturers.

CALIPER TECHNIQUE

The caliper technique for the estimation of body composition involves taking measurements of skin-fold thickness at various sites. These measurements are used in various equations to predict body fat. Due to its ease of use, measurement of skin-fold thickness is one of the most commonly used techniques to measure body fat. The technique is based on the assumption that the subcutaneous adipose layer reflects total body fat, but this association may vary with age and gender.

NOTE: Based on research, the most accurate methods of measuring body fat are hydrostatic weighing, Bod Pod, and body scan. Hydrostatic weighing, body scan, and high-end bioelectrical impedance machines are offered at many gyms and private health centers across the country. Do a simple search online, or ask around at your local gym. Another accurate measure of body fat is being tested with calipers by a professional certified in fitness testing. The most convenient method is to purchase a foot pad scale that you can use in your home and measure on a

BODY COMPOSITION ASSESSMENT

	START	3 WEEKS	6 WEEKS	9 WEEKS	12 WEEKS	15 WEEKS	18 WEEKS	21 WEEKS	
Body Weight									
Body Mass Index									
Body Fat Percentage (using one or more of the following methods: bioelectrical impedance scale, Bod Pod, body scan, caliper technique)									
Method 1									
Method 2									
Body Circumference Measurements									
Upper Arm (circumference) 1. Right									
2. Left									
Upper Thigh (circumference) 3. Right									
4. Left									
Mid-thigh (circumference) 5. Right									
6. Left									
7. Chest (at nipple line)									
8. Neck (middle)									
9. Hips (around highest peak of buttocks when standing with heels together)									
10. Waist (at belly button)									
11. Waist (at smallest point)									
Total body measurement (1–11)									

Form 4: Body Composition Assessment

24 WEEKS	27 WEEKS	30 WEEKS	33 WEEKS	36 WEEKS	39 WEEKS	42 WEEKS	45 WEEKS	48 WEEKS	52 WEEKS

regular basis without being inconvenienced. The important factor is that you remeasure using the same method and the same device.

BODY CIRCUMFERENCES

Getting a thorough sense of the size of your body is another useful set of parameters with which to monitor your progress. As you begin to decrease your body fat percentage and increase your lean muscle percentage, depending on your preexisting level of fitness, you may not see dramatic movement on the scale. In fact, it's possible to go down three whole clothing sizes, and lose only five or ten pounds. So to help you track your progress more accurately, and to keep you motivated when the scale just isn't making sense, get out a tape measure and take the following circumference measurements listed in Form 4. (According to the American Council of Sports Medicine, a waist girth measurement of greater than 35 inches for women, or 40 inches for men, indicates an increased risk of health complications, and a real need for weight loss.)

NOTE: Make sure to measure at the same spot when you repeat to track your progress.

Photocopy or download Form 4: Body Composition Assessment from www.theholly woodtrainer.com and follow the instructions for taking your body measurements. Put your completed form in the Measurements section of your journal.

GENETICS AND BODY TYPE

Before we talk about how to change your body, let's address the issue of what you *can't* change, so that you know what you can and cannot expect from this program. Each of us is a unique individual with our own genetic makeup, and this uniqueness extends to the basic shape of our bodies. In the 1940s, Dr. William Sheldon (1898–1977), an American psychologist who devoted his life to observing the variety of human bodies and temperaments, introduced the theory of different body types. He taught and did research at a number of American universities and is best known for his series of books on the human constitution. He described three basic body types: endomorph, mesomorph, and ectomorph. In fact, most people are a combination of two of these types, such as ecto-mesomorph, or endo-mesomorph.

Endomorph: This type is physically characterized by a generally soft body, tending to be rotund with underdeveloped muscles, having an overdeveloped digestive system and trouble losing weight, but gaining muscle easily. The personality traits associated with an endomorph are: love of food, tolerance, evenness of emotions, love of comfort, sociability, good humor, relaxed personality, and a need for affection.

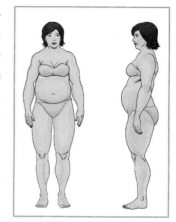

Mesomorph: This is the athletic body that tends to be husky and muscular, with upright posture and thick skin. The typical mesomorph shape is an hourglass in women and rectangular in men. Mesomorphs gain and lose weight easily and develop muscle quickly. They have a mature appearance early in life. The personality traits associated with a mesomorph are: adventurousness, a desire for power and dominance, courageousness, indifference to what others think or want, assertiveness, boldness, zest for physical activity, competitiveness, and a love of risk and chance.

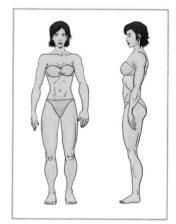

Ectomorph: Thin, flat-chested, and delicate in build, the typical ectomorph has a young appearance. The ectomorph tends to be tall, stoop-shouldered, and lightly muscled, with a large brain. Ectomorphs have trouble gaining weight and difficulty developing muscle. The personality traits associated with an ectomorph are: self-consciousness, a preference for privacy, an introverted nature, inhibition, social anxiousness, an artistic nature, mental intensity, and an emotionally restrained nature.

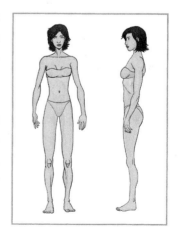

Once you've identified your body type, or the combination that best describes you, it is time to love your body. You can aesthetically change your body by losing or gaining fat and muscle in different areas of your body, but you will never completely change your body type. It's important to understand this because your weight-loss goals must be realistic.

It's vital to accept your body type for what it is so that you can start working toward becoming the best you that you can be—a beautiful, healthy representative of your type. Serena Williams is a mesomorph, Halle Berry an ectomorph. Both are healthy, beautiful women, and typical of their types. But even if they were on the same exercise and nutrition plans, they would never achieve the same bodies.

Despite the many claims, there is absolutely no evidence that exercise and weight loss are body-type specific. You cannot assume similarities between two people who have the same body type—the human body is simply too complex to be slotted into one of three general categories. It is more appropriate to prescribe exercise and nutrition based on your health screen, fitness assessment, and personal health and fitness goals. I want you to know your body type so you can accept yourself for who you are. Having a negative body image will often lead to lack of self-confidence, eating disorders, drug use (steroids, diet pills), surgery, and self-hatred.

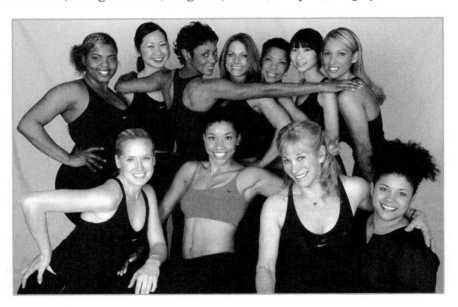

It is time to accept your specific body type and love the beautiful features that you do have. To help you find your individual beauty and confidence there is a positive quote and an affirmation at the beginning of each day in the twenty-one-day plan. So watch out—by the end of the three weeks you'll be ready to shine! If you feel you need some additional help in fighting a negative body image or eating disorder, here are some Internet resources to check out: www.lovemybody.org, www.bodypositive.com, www.bodyimagehealth.org, and www.pale-reflections.com.

CALORIES IN, CALORIES OUT

HOW MANY CALORIES A DAY DO YOU BURN?

I'm sure you know how much gas it takes to fill the tank of your car. But do you know how many calories your body needs to fill its "tank"? Overfill a gas tank and it'll just spill onto the ground, but do the same to your body and you get excess body fat. It's crucial to know your cutoff point so you can make sure you're not overfilling.

In order to calculate the total number of calories you burn in a day, also known as your total daily energy expenditure (TDEE), use the widely accepted Harris-Benedict Formula, which calculates your TDEE by first establishing the number of calories you would burn in a day doing absolutely nothing, simply maintaining basic body functions. This number, known as your basal metabolic rate (BMR), is a factor of your height, weight, and age.

To calculate your basal metabolic rate:

WOMEN

$$655 + (9.6 \times \text{weight in kg}) + (1.8 \times \text{height in cm}) - (4.7 \times \text{age})$$

MEN

$$66 + (13.7 \times \text{weight in kg}) + (5 \times \text{height in cm}) - (6.8 \times \text{age})$$

EXAMPLE:

A 30-year-old female weighing 180 lbs (81.8 kg) at 5'6" (167.6 cm):

$$\text{BMR} = 655 + (9.6 \times 81.8) + (1.8 \times 167.6) - (4.7 \times 30)$$

$$\text{BMR} = 655 + 785 + 302 - 141 = 1{,}601 \text{ calories/day}$$

NOTE: To convert pounds to kilograms divide by 2.2; to convert inches to centimeters multiply by 2.54.

To calculate your total daily energy expenditure (TDEE), start with your BMR. The Harris-Benedict Formula provides you with activity multipliers that assume five basic levels of daily physical activity. Multiply your BMR by the activity multiplier that best describes your daily level of physical activity to calculate your TDEE.

ACTIVITY MULTIPLIERS

1.2—Sedentary: you hold a desk job and get little or no exercise.

1.375—Light activity: you hold a desk job that requires light activity, or you exercise/play sports 1 to 3 days a week.

1.55—Moderate activity: you exercise/play sports 3 to 5 days a week.

1.725—Very active: you exercise/play sports 6 to 7 days a week.

1.9—Extra active: your job involves heavy physical activity, or you work out 2 or more times a day 3 or more days a week.

EXAMPLE:

BMR of 1,601 calories per day with sedentary activity (1.2).

TDEE: $1{,}601 \times 1.2 = 1{,}921$ calories/day

Once you know how many calories you burn in a day, it's easy to figure out the number of calories you can consume in your daily meal plan and the number of calories you need to burn

The Harris-Benedict Formula is very useful when it comes to calculating your total daily energy expenditure on your own, but it's important to remember that it is only an estimate, and can be up to 400 calories off. For the most accurate measure of your BMR, visit your health-care provider, who can test you based on your actual metabolism, rather than an equation. To prepare for this test you will be required to fast from midnight the night before. The test, which must be conducted first thing in the morning, requires that you sit very still in a Zen-like state and breathe into a mask that measures the amounts of oxygen and carbon dioxide in each breath. The information is recorded over 6 to 10 minutes, and then processed using an equation called the respiratory quotient to determine your personal BMR. The average cost of having this test done is between $35 and $80. To find a health-care center, gym, or other facility near you that offers this test go to www.newleaffitness.com or call 1-888-826-2751.

during your workouts in order to shed body fat. For example, to shed one pound of fat, you need to burn an extra 3,500 calories. So in order to lose two pounds a week (a healthy goal to set), you need to burn an excess of 7,000 calories a week.

There are two factors that you can control to help you lose body fat: the amount of physical activity you do (calories burned/output) and the amount of food you eat (calorie intake). Following (in Form 5) are three different Daily Calorie Intake and Output charts to help you plan and organize the number of calories you can eat in your daily meal plan and the amount of exercise required for you to burn that fat. In the twenty-one-day plan, outlined in Part 5, I have provided you with complete daily meal plans, and by using these charts in conjunction with the meal plan you can create the exact portion sizes that work for your goals. These charts are extremely important in providing you the flexibility you need to be successful in the real world. Each person who uses the plan is going to have his or her own specific total daily energy expenditure because of individual height and weight. Some days you might only be able to fit in a 20-minute workout instead of 30 minutes, in which case you may burn only 200 calories in your workout, but you can adjust your food intake so that you can still reach your goal. The important thing to note is that you should never, ever take in fewer than 1,200 calories a day. Research shows that when you consume less than that your body goes into starvation mode, and it will hold on to your body fat because it is afraid that you will not eat enough calories. Remember our history: we used to be hunters and gatherers, and our genetics are designed for survival.

Therefore, we have specific mechanisms that kick into action when our body is in fear of not getting enough food. Your body will burn fewer calories and conserve as much as it can in order to survive. Keep eating and you will keep burning.

Of the three Daily Calorie Intake and Output charts that appear in Form 5, following, the first is for burning 2 pounds a week; the second is for burning 1.5 pounds a week; and the third is for burning 1 pound a week. These are provided as guidelines only. You can modify any of the charts to work with your specific weekly schedule. Just make sure the weekly total for the number of calories burned is accurate: $-7,000$ for 2 pounds, $-5,250$ for 1.5 pounds, and $-3,500$ for 1 pound.

Here is an example of a completed Daily Calorie Intake and Output chart (to lose 1.5 pounds per week) based on the same thirty-year-old female we used to calculate total daily energy expenditure.

A 30-year-old female weighing 180 pounds (81.8 kg) at 5'6" (167.6 cm):
BMR $= 655 + 785 + 302 - 141 = 1,601$ calories/day
Activity (sedentary): 1.2
TDEE: $1,601 \times 1.2 = 1,921$ calories/day

1. TDEE appears in the chart with a negative sign, representing calories expended.
2. Number of calories burned during workouts, which is 300 on average and can be higher depending on height, intensity of workout, and muscle mass. To put in exact calorie output, a heart rate monitor used during workout sessions calculates calorie expenditure.
3. Add TDEE (1,921) and exercise calories burned in one day (300), which is 2,221 calories. This means 2,221 calories will be leaving the body as calories burned.
4. Subtract desired total calorie negative at the end of the day, which is 800 for Monday through Saturday ($2,221 - 800 = 1,421$ calories). This means one can eat 1,421 calories Monday through Saturday. For Sunday, the resting day instead of exercising, take the TDEE of 1,921 calories and subtract 450 calories, which is the desired total daily negative at the end of the day, which leaves 1,471 calories that you can eat on Sunday. You can adjust the calorie intake and output chart to fit your specific goals and your weekly schedule.

	MONDAY	TUESDAY	WEDNESDAY	THURSDAY	FRIDAY	SATURDAY	SUNDAY
EXAMPLE OF COMPLETED DAILY CALORIE INTAKE AND OUTPUT CHART TO LOSE 1.5 POUNDS PER WEEK							
−TDEE	−1,921	−1,921	−1,921	−1,921	−1,921	−1,921	−1,921
+FOOD	+1,421	+1,421	+1,421	+1,421	+1,421	+1,421	+1,471
−EXERCISE	−300	−300	−300	−300	−300	−300	REST
TOTAL (−5,250)	−800	−800	−800	−800	−800	−800	−450

> Photocopy or download Form 5, follow the instructions in Chapter 6 to determine your basal metabolic rate (BMR) and total daily energy expenditure (TDEE)—the number of calories you burn in a day—and place the completed form in the Measurements section of your journal.

1. Place your calculated TDEE in every day of the chart.
2. Place the calories that you plan to burn on each day that you plan to work out. On your day of rest there should be a 0 in the exercise column. The average number of calories burned using the Hollywood Trainer Workouts in this book is 300 calories per 30 minutes. Keep in mind that some people will burn slightly more or less due to individual metabolism, muscle mass, height, weight, effort, and intensity throughout the workout. For the purpose of this chart, it is sufficient to put 300 calories as an average.
3. Now that you have the TDEE (metabolism) and your desired exercise calorie output in the chart for each day, add them together for the total calories leaving your body each day (from metabolism and exercise).
4. Subtract your desired daily calorie negative total (1,100, 800, 500) from the total daily calories leaving your body (total from number 3) and you will have the total daily food calories that you can consume. Figure out this number for each day and place it in the food column to complete each day. This is the number of calories that you can eat each day. Place this number at the top of your Daily Food Log.

DAILY CALORIE INTAKE AND OUTPUT CHARTS

My basal metabolic rate (BMR): _____ (calories a day)

My total daily energy expenditure (TDEE): _____ (calories a day)

DAILY CALORIE INTAKE AND OUTPUT CHART (FOR LOSING 2 POUNDS A WEEK)

	Monday	Tuesday	Wednesday	Thursday	Friday	Saturday	Sunday
−TDEE							
+Food							
−Exercise							
Total (−7,000)	−1,100	−1,100	−1,100	−1,100	−1,100	−1,100	−400

DAILY CALORIE INTAKE AND OUTPUT CHART (FOR LOSING 1.5 POUNDS A WEEK)

	Monday	Tuesday	Wednesday	Thursday	Friday	Saturday	Sunday
−TDEE							
+Food							
−Exercise							
Total (−5,250)	−800	−800	−800	−800	−800	−800	−450

DAILY CALORIE INTAKE AND OUTPUT CHART (FOR LOSING 1 POUND A WEEK)

	Monday	Tuesday	Wednesday	Thursday	Friday	Saturday	Sunday
−TDEE							
+Food							
−Exercise							
Total (−3,500)	−500	−500	−500	−500	−500	−500	−500

Form 5: Daily Calorie Intake and Output Charts

YOUR PERSONAL FITNESS PROFILE

The only thing that remains for you to find out about your body before you launch into the program is how fit you are right now. Assessing your current level of fitness is important not only as a baseline comparison against which to measure your progress, but also because my exercise plan accounts for twelve different levels of fitness, and if you're going to get the most out of the program, it's important to know where to start. Your personal fitness profile will be determined by the following tests: cardiorespiratory fitness; muscular endurance: abdominals and lower body; muscular strength: abdominals and upper body; and flexibility. Once you've completed all the tests, fill out the form at the end of this section and put it in the Measurements section of your journal.

CARDIORESPIRATORY FITNESS TESTS

VO2MAX AND YOUR TARGET HEART RATE TRAINING ZONES
Cardiorespiratory fitness is your body's ability to transport oxygen and blood to your working muscles for a prolonged period (12 minutes or more). The term *cardiorespiratory fitness* is often

used interchangeably with *aerobic fitness*. *Aerobic* literally means "with oxygen," and refers to the use of oxygen in *muscles'* energy-generating process.

There are many ways of testing your level of cardiorespiratory fitness, both at home and with the help of a fitness or health-care professional. Although it is not compulsory as it is in the case of checking blood pressure or cholesterol, a visit to a health-care professional in order to establish your level of cardio fitness or your target heart rate zones is recommended. Any information you get from a professional test will usually be more accurate and reliable than that from a self-test. A cardiorespiratory test—also known as a stress test, an aerobic test, or a VO2 sub-max test—administered by a fitness or health-care professional will cost between $50 and $200. These tests will provide you the following valuable information:

Cardiorespiratory Fitness Level: how you compare to the rest of your age group.

Anaerobic Threshold: the heart rate level at which you stop using fat as a fuel source and use 100 percent sugars.

Caloric Burn Rate: the number of calories you burn in a minute of exercise, what percentage of that number is from fat, and what percentage is from sugar.

Breathing Rate and Quality: Do you inhale large volumes of oxygen with every breath, or do you hyperventilate or take small, shallow breaths? (Oxygen is needed at the cellular level to burn fat; therefore, how you breathe and how much oxygen you bring into your body are good things to know.)

True Heart-Rate Training Zones: There are generic formulas that help you figure out your own heart rate training zones, but they will only give you a general estimate. By having a professionally administered cardio test, you are guaranteed that the results are based on your unique fitness level and your body, and are therefore more accurate than the results of any formulaic calculations.

VO2max: the maximum amount of oxygen that can be used by the body for maximal sustained exercise. Since the body uses oxygen to convert food (fat) into energy, the more oxygen you can consume, the more energy, power, or speed you can produce, and the more calories you can burn.

To find a cardio testing center in your area, visit www.newleaffitness.com, call your local gym, university, or health-care center, or do a search online. Remember, there are several names for the same test: VO2 sub-max test, active metabolic test, aerobic test, stress test, cardiorespiratory test, step test, walking test, among others. Make sure you can see an example of the printout of information that the test will provide so you can determine whether it will be valuable information for you. The main purpose of this test is to determine your cardiovascular condition, which involves the condition and capability of your heart and lungs.

ROCKPORT FITNESS WALKING TEST

If it is not possible for you to get a test administered by a professional, there are still ways to get some of the vital information you need about your cardiorespiratory fitness before you get started on the exercise program. The one that I think is most convenient is the Rockport Fitness Walking Test.

For this test you are asked to walk one mile as fast as you can, and then to record your heart rate as soon as you've finished, as well as the time it took you to complete the mile. (I don't want to hear any excuses about not being able to figure out how far a mile is—use a premeasured walking path or a high-school track, or measure a route using the odometer on your car.) To take your pulse immediately after walking a mile, count beats at the carotid artery (your neck) for 15 seconds, then multiply by 4. Even better, you can wear a heart rate monitor.

Rockport Fitness Walking Test Results:

My body weight (BW): _____

My age (A): _____

My gender (G) (0 for female, 1 for male): _____

My time to walk one mile (T): _____

My heart rate immediately after walking one mile (HR): _____

VO2MAX

By plugging the information derived from the Rockport Fitness Walking Test into the formula below, you get an accurate prediction of your VO2max, or the point at which your oxygen intake is at its peak. VO2max is one of the best indicators of cardiorespiratory fitness.

$$VO2max = 132.853 - (0.0769 \times BW) - (0.3877 \times A) +$$
$$(6.315 \times G) - (3.2649 \times T) - (0.1565 \times HR)$$

Example: You walked one mile in 15.75 minutes and your heart rate at the end of that mile was 155 beats per minute. You are a thirty-two-year-old woman who weighs 180 pounds. Therefore, your VO2max formula looks like this:

$$132.853 - (0.0769 \times 180) - (0.3877 \times 32) +$$
$$(6.315 \times 0) - (3.2649 \times 15.75) - (0.1565 \times 155) =$$
$$132.853 - 13.842 - 12.406 + 0 - 51.422 - 24.258 = 30.925$$

VO2max score of 30.925 for a thirty-two-year-old woman

VO2max rating of fair

Once you've established your VO2max, see where you rate according to the following table. As you work out on a regular basis, your VO2max can improve. Remember that this number is the maximum amount of oxygen that can be used by your body for maximal sustained exercise. This oxygen is necessary to turn fat and sugar into energy so you can burn it off. The more your VO2max improves, the more oxygen you can bring into your body, and the better you become at breaking down fat and sugar and burning them off as fuel.

VO2MAX RATINGS

WOMEN

Rating	Score				
	(AGES 20–29)	(AGES 30–39)	(AGES 40–49)	(AGES 50–59)	(AGES 60–69)
LOW	Below 28	Below 27	Below 25	Below 21	Below 16
FAIR	29–34	28–32	26–30	22–27	17–22
AVERAGE	35–43	33–41	31–39	28–36	23–30
GOOD	44–48	42–47	40–44	37–41	31–36
EXCELLENT	Over 48	Over 47	Over 44	Over 41	Over 37

(continued)

MEN					
	(AGES 20–29)	(AGES 30–39)	(AGES 40–49)	(AGES 50–59)	(AGES 60–69)
LOW	Below 37	Below 34	Below 30	Below 24	Below 21
FAIR	38–43	35–38	31–35	25–30	22–26
AVERAGE	44–51	39–47	36–43	31–38	27–35
GOOD	52–56	48–51	44–46	39–43	36–38
EXCELLENT	Over 56	Over 51	Over 46	Over 43	Over 38

Table 1

YOUR VO2

VO2max Score: _____

VO2max Rating: _____

Have a look at the VO2max numbers of some athletes:

General Population, Female, Ages 20–29: 35–43 ml/kg/min

General Population, Male, Ages 20–29: 44–51

U.S. College Track, Male: 57.4

College Students, Male: 44.6

Highest Recorded Female (cross-country skier): 74

Highest Recorded Male (cross-country skier): 94

Lance Armstrong, professional cyclist: 83.7

Greg LeMond, professional cyclist: 92.5

Frank Shorter, U.S. Olympic marathon winner: 71.3

Ingrid Kristiansen, ex-marathon world record holder: 71.2

Rosa Mota, marathon runner: 67.2

Derek Clayton, Australian ex-marathon world record holder: 69.7

Jarmila Kratochvílová, Czech Olympian 400m/800m winner: 72.8

HEART-RATE TRAINING ZONES

Fitness experts and coaches have figured out that each one of us has an ideal heart rate for training that is going to help us achieve maximum results. It is important to distinguish your heart rate training zones so that you can get the most out of your workout. Time is your most valuable commodity, so let's make sure that you are working out smart and getting the most effective and efficient workout to achieve your particular goals. By establishing your heart rate training zones, and by monitoring your heart rate during exercise, you will be able to effectively monitor your progress so you can continue to push yourself to the next level. If you can't get a professionally administered cardiorespiratory test, the next best thing is to use a heart rate max formula. A few different formulas are available, but I have chosen the Simple Heart Rate Max Formula because it is easy to use and the only number you need to know is your age. Your maximum heart rate is an estimation of the maximum number of beats that your heart will beat in one minute. Once you have determined your maximum heart rate by using the simple formula you can determine your heart-rate training zones. Training zones are important not only for effective training but also for your safety. The following are examples of people who would benefit from heart-rate training zones:

1. New exercisers, who don't know how hard to push themselves. Some overdo it and get injured; others don't push themselves hard enough, ending up with poor results.
2. Exercisers who are recovering from surgery or under strict guidelines from their doctor.
3. Exercisers who are pregnant.
4. Exercisers who want to get the most out of every workout and don't have time to waste guessing whether they are working at the right intensity.

The following formula calculates your heart rate max according to your age. It is *only* an estimate.

Heart rate max = 220 − your age

Example: thirty-five-year-old female or male, 220 − 35 = 185 bpm

Heart rate max for someone who is thirty-five years old is 185 bpm.

Your heart rate max = _____ bpm

CALCULATE YOUR ESTIMATED HEART RATE TRAINING ZONES

If you get a cardiorespiratory fitness test, then you will receive exact training zones based on your metabolic profile and VO2max from whoever administers your test. If you cannot get a professional cardio test, you will need to approximate your heart rate zones for the following levels of intensity, all of which you will need to get the most out of my exercise program.

Here are a few zones of particular importance to you as you start the program:

Aerobic Base Training Zone: 60 to 75 Percent Heart Rate Max: Your aerobic base is the heart rate range where you can exercise comfortably for long periods of time (20 to 60 minutes or more) without stopping. When you first start exercising, your heart rate will skyrocket to 75 percent or more because your body is not used to exercising. Your heart has to work very hard to circulate your blood to your muscles, where it is needed. As you become consistent in exercising and your body more conditioned, your heart rate will not increase as much when completing the same exercises. When your heart rate stays at 50 to 60 percent of your heart rate max for the entire length of your cardio workout, then it is time to take it to the next level. Aerobic base training is the most important zone for a new exerciser.

The more you condition your aerobic base, the more you will improve and strengthen your heart and lungs. You will find it easier to function in everyday life, without running out of breath or energy, and you will improve your oxygen consumption, which will help you burn more fat. In addition, conditioning your aerobic base will make it easier for you to complete circuit training, weight training, and other types of sports. Having a conditioned aerobic base will also

---

Your aerobic base training zone: _____ bpm

Example: aerobic base training zone, 60–75 percent of 185 bpm, which is the heart rate max of a 35-year-old female or male, is calculated as:

$$0.60 \times 185 \text{ bpm for the low limit} = 111 \text{ bpm}$$
$$.75 \times 185 \text{ bpm for the high limit} = 139 \text{ bpm}$$

The aerobic base training zone for a 35-year-old female or male using the simple formula is 111–139 bpm.

help you recover better in between weight-training exercises. Every great fitness program starts with conditioning the aerobic base. The twelve-level cardio program in the exercise section and the twenty-one-day plan of this book are going to help you.

Intermediate-to-Advanced Aerobic Training Zone: 65 to 85 Percent Heart Rate Max: As you progress with your workouts, your heart, lungs, oxygen consumption, and muscular endurance all will improve. After a while, working out in your base training zone will not be challenging to you. When this happens, you'll want to up the intensity to 65 to 85 percent of your heart rate max. Make sure when you increase intensity that you can still complete the exercises feeling good and maintaining good form. If you can, then you're going to be burning more calories and conditioning your body at a higher level. You should be able to carry on a conversation or talk for 15- to 20-second intervals to be successfully training your aerobic base at an intermediate to advanced level.

Interval Aerobic Training Zone: 70 to 90 Percent Heart Rate Max: This is the target zone for all levels of exercisers when doing short (anywhere from 15 seconds to 3 minutes), high-intensity intervals. Interval training is a form of training that alternates bouts of heavy or very heavy work with periods of rest or light work. The two circuits and the cardio program in the exercise section all contain interval training. Interval training that consists of alternating between weights and cardio movements is a great way of creating time-saving, effective workouts. You get the best of both worlds in one short, energizing session. Not only does interval training save you time, but studies show that high-intensity training continues to elevate your

Your intermediate-to-advanced aerobic training zone is: _____ bpm
Example: intermediate-to-advanced aerobic training zone, 65–85 percent of 185 bpm, which is the heart-rate max of a 35-year-old female or male, is calculated as:

$$.65 \times 185 \text{ bpm for the low limit} = 120 \text{ bpm}$$
$$.85 \times 185 \text{ bpm for the high limit} = 157 \text{ bpm}$$

The intermediate-to-advanced aerobic training zone for a 35-year-old male or female using the simple formula is 120–157 bpm.

metabolic rate and oxygen consumption after you are finished exercising for anywhere from 15 minutes to 48 hours, which means that you continue to burn calories and fat at higher rates even after your workout is complete. This is known as "after burn," or EPOC (excess postexercise oxygen consumption). And since your heart rate is higher, you will also be burning more calories during the workout. Most of the calories you will burn *during* the workout will use sugar stores rather than fat reserves (sugar being the more readily available energy source). But don't be concerned because you will continue to burn fat at higher rates after your high-intensity workout than you would burn during a low-intensity workout of the same duration.

Your interval training zone is: _____ bpm

Example: interval training zone, 70–90 percent of 185 bpm, which is the heart rate max of a 35-year-old female or male, is calculated as:

$$.70 \times 185 \text{ bpm for the low limit} = 130 \text{ bpm}$$
$$.90 \times 185 \text{ bpm for the high limit} = 167 \text{ bpm}$$

The interval training zone for a 35-year-old male or female using the simple formula is 130–167 bpm.

MONITORING YOUR HEART RATE

The best way to monitor your heart rate during a workout is simply to use a heart rate monitor. Available at any sporting-goods store, my favorites are the Nike Triax c6 or the Nike Imara, and the Polar F4, F6, or F11, but there are several models for you to choose from. A good monitor will allow you to input your age, height, and weight, and will then tell you how many calories you are burning during your workout, as well as how fast your heart is beating.

The low-tech option for monitoring your heart rate is to take your pulse manually during your workout. Place your index and middle fingers at your carotid (neck) or radial (wrist) artery, and count the number of beats in 6 seconds, then add a zero to get your beats per minute (bpm). It's best to take your pulse 2 to 3 times during a workout, to make sure you are hitting your proper training zones.

Forms 8 and 9 in the Appendix are your Cardiorespiratory Training Log and your Circuit Training Log master sheets. These forms should be photocopied and put into the Exercise section of your journal. Throughout your workouts you are asked to record your heart rate at specific points so you can monitor your progress and determine when it is time to challenge yourself to reach the next level.

MUSCULAR ENDURANCE TEST: ABDOMINALS

Muscular endurance provides you with the ability to do several repetitions of a movement or to hold a particular position for an extended amount of time without injuring yourself or becoming fatigued. Muscular endurance is required to do basic everyday functions for long periods of time like sitting upright at your desk, walking, or standing up with good posture. If you are weak in muscular endurance you will often compensate with other muscle groups and create chronic injuries. Muscular strength is necessary for strong or explosive movements like lifting a box or luggage, catching yourself if you slip or fall, lifting your children, or pushing or pulling your body from a place of danger to one of safety when in an accident. People who are lacking in muscular strength will often injure themselves when trying to execute any of the above.

Testing your abdominal endurance is a simple matter of counting how many sit-ups you can do in one minute. The sit-ups should be performed as follows: lying faceup on the floor with knees

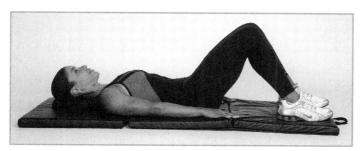

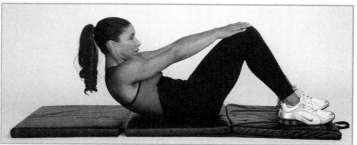

MUSCULAR ENDURANCE TEST: ABDOMINALS SCORES AND RATINGS

WOMEN

Rating	Score					
	(AGES 18–25)	(AGES 26–35)	(AGES 36–45)	(AGES 46–55)	(AGES 56–65)	(AGES 65+)
VERY POOR	Less than 18	Less than 13	Less than 7	Less than 5	Less than 3	Less than 2
POOR	18–24	13–20	7–14	5–9	3–6	2–4
BELOW AVERAGE	25–28	21–24	15–18	10–13	7–9	5–10
AVERAGE	29–32	25–28	19–22	14–17	10–12	11–13
ABOVE AVERAGE	33–36	29–32	23–26	18–21	13–17	14–16
GOOD	37–43	33–39	27–33	22–27	18–24	17–23
EXCELLENT	More than 43	More than 39	More than 33	More than 27	More than 24	More than 23

MEN

Rating	(AGES 18–25)	(AGES 26–35)	(AGES 36–45)	(AGES 46–55)	(AGES 56–65)	(AGES 65+)
VERY POOR	Less than 25	Less than 22	Less than 17	Less than 13	Less than 9	Less than 7
POOR	25–30	22–28	17–22	13–17	9–12	7–10
BELOW AVERAGE	31–34	29–30	23–26	18–21	13–16	11–14
AVERAGE	35–38	31–34	27–29	22–24	17–20	15–18
ABOVE AVERAGE	39–43	35–39	30–34	25–28	21–24	19–21
GOOD	44–49	40–45	35–41	29–35	25–31	22–28
EXCELLENT	More than 49	More than 45	More than 41	More than 35	More than 31	More than 28

(Source: adapted from *Y's Way to Physical Fitness*, Lawrence A. Golding, et al., 1986)
Table 2

bent and feet flat on the ground shoulder width apart, and hands resting on the floor, slowly squeeze your stomach, pushing the small of your back flat into the floor, and lift yourself up until your hands touch the top of your knees. Do not pull yourself up using your head or neck, and keep your lower back on the floor at all times. (You do not need to come to a full sitting position.) Time yourself for one minute and see how you rate according to Table 2.

Muscular Endurance Test: Abdominals Score: _____

Muscular Endurance Rating: Abdominals Rating: _____

MUSCULAR ENDURANCE TEST: LOWER BODY

To test your lower body muscular endurance, perform leg squats until the point of exhaustion. Stand in front of a chair or bench as though you are about to sit on it, with your feet slightly wider than shoulder width apart. (The best size chair to use is one that makes a right angle of your knees when you are seated comfortably in it.) Squat down until your butt just grazes the seat of the chair or bench, but stand back up before you rest any weight on it. Keep your back straight and perform the movements without jerking. Repeat until you are fatigued. Record your number of squats (score) and see how you perform against the accepted standards outlined in Table 3.

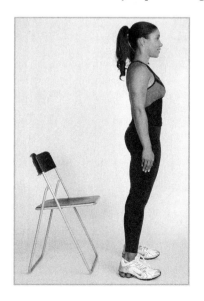
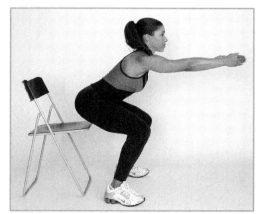

MUSCULAR ENDURANCE TEST: LOWER BODY SCORES AND RATINGS

WOMEN

Rating	Score					
	(AGES 18-25)	(AGES 26-35)	(AGES 36-45)	(AGES 46-55)	(AGES 56-65)	(AGES 65+)
VERY POOR	0–17	0–12	0–6	0–4	0–2	0–1
POOR	18–24	13–20	7–14	5–9	3–6	2–4
BELOW AVERAGE	25–28	21–24	15–18	10–13	7–9	5–10
AVERAGE	29–32	25–28	19–22	14–17	10–12	11–13
ABOVE AVERAGE	33–36	29–32	23–26	18–21	13–17	14–16
GOOD	37–43	33–39	27–33	22–27	18–24	17–23
EXCELLENT	More than 43	More than 39	More than 33	More than 27	More than 24	More than 23

MEN

Rating	Score					
	(AGES 18-25)	(AGES 26-35)	(AGES 36-45)	(AGES 46-55)	(AGES 56-65)	(AGES 65+)
VERY POOR	0–24	0–21	0–16	0–12	0–8	0–6
POOR	25–30	22–28	17–22	13–17	9–12	7–10
BELOW AVERAGE	31–34	29–30	23–26	18–21	13–16	11–14
AVERAGE	35–38	31–34	27–29	22–24	17–20	15–18
ABOVE AVERAGE	39–43	35–39	30–34	25–28	21–24	19–21
GOOD	44–49	40–45	35–41	29–35	25–31	22–28
EXCELLENT	More than 49	More than 45	More than 41	More than 35	More than 31	More than 28

(Source: adapted from *Y's Way to Physical Fitness*, Lawrence A. Golding, et al., 1986)
Table 3

Muscular Endurance Test: Lower Body Score: _____

Muscular Endurance Rating: Lower Body Rating: _____

MUSCULAR STRENGTH: ABDOMINALS

To test your abdominal strength, complete one sit-up at seven progressive levels of difficulty. The highest level at which you can complete one sit-up is your score. Begin in the basic sit-up starting position: lie faceup with legs bent at the knees, feet flat on the ground about shoulder width apart. Follow the instructions in the chart below, as shown in the photos following.

MUSCULAR STRENGTH TEST: ABDOMINALS SCORE, RATING, AND PERFORMANCE DESCRIPTION

Score	Rating	Performance Description
0	VERY POOR	Cannot perform one sit-up
1	POOR	With arms at your sides, lift yourself up until your wrists are level with your thighs.
2	FAIR	With arms at your sides, lift yourself up until your elbows are level with your thighs.
3	AVERAGE	With your hands crossed at your abs, lift yourself up until your chest is level with your thighs.
4	GOOD	With your hands across your chest, lift yourself up until your forearms are level with your thighs.
5	VERY GOOD	With your hands behind your head and elbows out, lift yourself up until your chest is level with your thighs.
6	EXCELLENT	Holding a 5-pound weight behind your head, lift yourself up until your chest is level with your thighs.
7	ELITE	Holding a 10-pound weight behind your head, lift yourself up until your chest is level with your thighs.

(Source: adapted from *Y's Way to Physical Fitness*, Lawrence A. Golding, et al., 1986)
Table 4

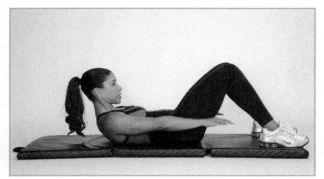

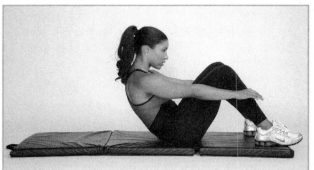

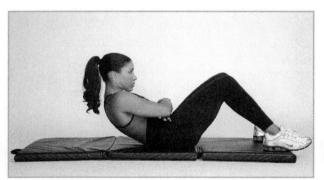

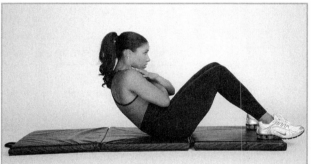

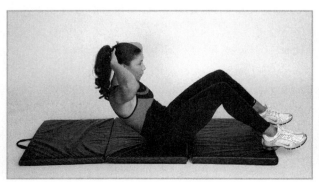

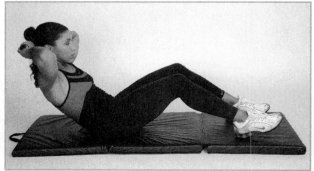

Muscular Strength Test: Abdominals Score: _____

Muscular Strength Rating: Abdominals Rating: _____

MUSCULAR STRENGTH: UPPER BODY

This test involves doing push-ups. For women, the accepted version uses the "bent knee" position, in which your hands, knees, and tops of the feet all touch the floor. For men, the standard is the "military style" push-up position, with only hands and toes touching the floor. Perform as many as you can without compromising form—your back should remain straight and you should move from a fully extended arm position until your nose just touches the floor. Perform a full push-up each time—until you reach exhaustion. Use Table 5 to see how you rate.

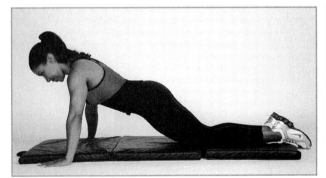
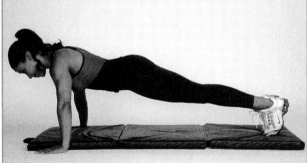
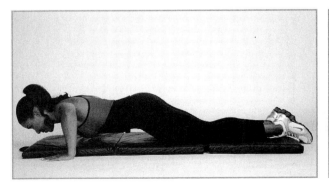
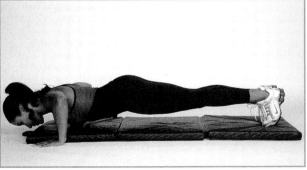

RATINGS FOR UPPER BODY STRENGTH TEST

WOMEN

Rating	Score					
	(AGES 17—19)	(AGES 20—29)	(AGES 30—39)	(AGES 40—49)	(AGES 50—59)	(AGES 60—65)
VERY POOR	0–1	0–1	0	0	0	0
POOR	2–5	2–6	1–4	1–3	1–2	1
BELOW AVERAGE	6–10	7–11	5–9	4–7	3–6	2–4
AVERAGE	11–20	12–22	10–21	8–17	7–14	5–12
ABOVE AVERAGE	21–27	23–29	22–30	18–24	15–20	13–18
GOOD	28–35	30–36	31–37	25–31	21–25	19–23
EXCELLENT	More than 35	More than 36	More than 37	More than 31	More than 25	More than 23

MEN

Rating	Score					
	(AGES 17-19)	(AGES 20-29)	(AGES 30-39)	(AGES 40-49)	(AGES 50-59)	(AGES 60-65)
VERY POOR	Less than 4	Less than 4	Less than 2	0	0	0
POOR	4–10	4–9	2–7	1–5	1–4	1–2
BELOW AVERAGE	11–18	10–16	8–12	6–10	5–8	3–5
AVERAGE	19–34	17–29	13–24	11–20	9–17	6–16
ABOVE AVERAGE	35–46	30–39	25–33	21–28	18–24	17–23
GOOD	47–56	40–47	34–41	29–34	25–31	24–30
EXCELLENT	More than 56	More than 47	More than 41	More than 34	More than 31	More than 30

(Source: adapted from *Y's Way to Physical Fitness*, Lawrence A. Golding, et al., 1986)
Table 5: Ratings for Upper Body Strength Test

Muscular Strength Test: Upper Body Score: _____

Muscular Strength Rating: Upper Body Rating: _____

FLEXIBILITY TEST

Ask a friend to help you with this one. Take off your shoes and sit on the floor with your legs straight out in front of you, with feet flexed so your toes are pointing toward the ceiling. With your arms extended in front of you, slowly and smoothly reach forward as far as you can without bending your knees and hold for a two-count stretch. Have your friend measure in millimeters how far beyond your toes (positive measurement) or how far short of your toes (negative measurement) you can reach. Do this twice, without any jerky movements, and record your best score. Check your score against expected standards in Table 6 to determine your personal rating.

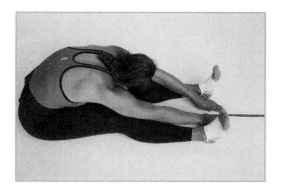
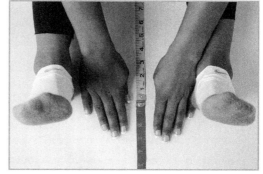

FLEXIBILITY SCORES AND RATINGS

Rating	Score	
	WOMEN (IN MM)	MEN (IN MM)
VERY POOR	More than −15	More than −20
POOR	−14 to −8	−19 to −9
FAIR	−7 to 0	−8 to −1
AVERAGE	1 to 10	0 to 5
GOOD	11 to 20	6 to 16
EXCELLENT	21 to 30	17 to 27
SUPER	Beyond 30	Beyond 27

(Source: adapted from *Y's Way to Physical Fitness*, Lawrence A. Golding, et al., 1986)
Table 6: Flexibility Scores and Ratings

Flexibility Test Score: _____ mm

Flexibility Test Rating: _____

Congratulations—you've completed the preliminary tests, forms, and questionnaires, and you definitely know a lot more about yourself now than you did when you started. Use the parameters to monitor your success as you move forward and start to transform your health. Before moving on to the Nutrition chapter, take some time to enter all of the measurements, rates, and scores into Your Personal Fitness Profile (Form 6), which follows. (Remember, you can photocopy this form or download it at www.thehollywoodtrainer.com and keep it in your journal.) Going forward, you can use this form to record your stats in three-week intervals. It will help keep you motivated as you watch your results and your measurements improve in the upcoming weeks.

BEFORE-AND-AFTER PHOTOS

Watch your body change as you change your life. Take four photos of yourself—front view, left side view, right side view, and back view—and paste them in the appropriate boxes of the Before-and-After Photos (Form 11), which is in the Appendix. Make sure that you are wearing a bathing suit, bikini, or formfitting workout bra and shorts. (If you cover yourself up, it will be more difficult to see the physical changes in your body; these are the changes that you will not see on the scale, but you will be amazed when you look back at your photos.) Photocopy the form and put it into the Measurements section of your journal. Continue to take new photos every six weeks and put them in your Measurements section.

YOUR PERSONAL FITNESS PROFILE

	START	3 WEEKS	6 WEEKS	9 WEEKS	12 WEEKS	15 WEEKS	18 WEEKS	21 WEEKS	
Resting Heart Rate									
Blood Pressure*									
LDL Cholesterol									
HDL Cholesterol									
Total Cholesterol*									
Triglycerides									
Body Weight									
Body Mass Index (BMI)									
Body Fat Percentage Method 1									
Method 2									
Upper Arm (circumference) 1. Right									
2. Left									
Upper Thigh (circumference) 3. Right									
4. Left									
Mid-thigh (circumference) 5. Right									
6. Left									
7. Chest (at nipple line)									
8. Neck (middle)									
9. Hips									
10. Waist (at belly button)									
11. Waist (at smallest point)									
Body Circumference Total									
VO2max score and rating from Cardiorespiratory Test or Rockport Fitness Walking Test									
Muscular Strength: Abs									
Muscular Strength: Upper Body									
Muscular Endurance: Abs									
Muscular Endurance: Lower Body									
Flexibility									

Form 6: Your Personal Fitness Profile

*Blood pressure and cholesterol levels need only be tested again after twelve weeks.

24 WEEKS	27 WEEKS	30 WEEKS	33 WEEKS	36 WEEKS	39 WEEKS	42 WEEKS	45 WEEKS	48 WEEKS	52 WEEKS

Part Three

21 DAYS THAT WILL
CHANGE YOUR LIFE

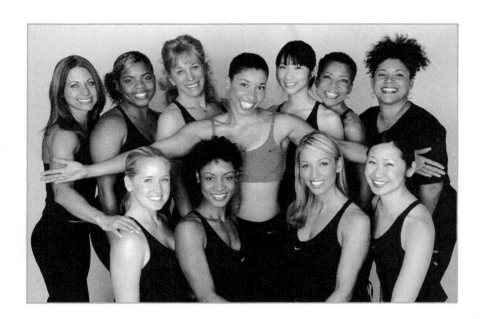

You've made it through all the prep work, and now you're ready for the twenty-one days that will change your life. For the next three weeks, the daily plans I've put together will guide you step by step, day by day, to a brand-new way of life. Each day begins with an inspirational message reflecting one of the seven principles for healthy living, followed by a daily menu, workout, testimonial, and exercise and nutrition tips so you can take control of your health—and your life—once and for all. What *you* do each day will determine your success. So keep a positive attitude—you *can* do this!

8

THE 21-DAY HOLLYWOOD TRAINER™ WEIGHT-LOSS PLAN

DAY 1

God helps those who help themselves.
—*Benjamin Franklin*

This is the beginning of a brand-new journey, an opportunity to change your habits, your body, and your life. First you must recognize and acknowledge the fact that you have everything you need to achieve the healthy body and full life that you want and deserve. Turn up that smile and fill your heart with joy—this is going to be a great day—the first of many to come.

> *Today's Affirmation*
> I already possess everything I need to succeed;
> there is nothing to stop me from reaching my goals.

10 THINGS TO KEEP YOU GOING

It's a tough world out there, and everyone needs to find sources of inspiration to fight off demons. Before you get started with your day, get out your journal and make a list of ten things that are your sources of joy and motivation. Whether it's a favorite saying, a photo, a person, or a place you love, your list should include things that nourish and inspire you, both mentally and spiritually. When you're having a tough day and you need that extra spark to get yourself ignited, you'll want to come back to this list—so make it a good list. You might also want to hang this list on your refrigerator or bulletin board as a daily reminder.

TODAY'S FOOD

WRITE IT DOWN

The first step to changing your eating habits is to be fully aware of what you eat. Using the Daily Food Log (Form 7), keep a daily record of your caloric intake, as well as a breakdown of how many grams of fat, protein, carbohydrates, fiber, sugar, and sodium you've had.

DAILY HYDRATION

Water is on the menu every day, and I recommend drinking half your body weight in ounces. This may sound like a lot, but if you keep water at hand throughout the day you won't have any problem getting proper hydration.

The Menu

Recipes marked with an asterisk (*) can be found in the recipe section, Chapter 17.

BREAKFAST: Berry Banana Oatmeal*, 1 hard-boiled egg, green tea or decaf coffee
SNACK: ½ cup organic low-fat cottage cheese with ½ cup fresh berries
LUNCH: Turkey Pita Sandwich *

SNACK: 1 orange
SNACK: 4 low-fat whole wheat crackers with 1 string organic low-fat cheese
DINNER: Broiled Honey-Mustard Salmon*/Broccoli Parmesan*/Honey-Glazed Carrots*
DESSERT: Chef Ronnda's Sexy Strawberry Walnut Dessert*
WATER: Half your body weight in ounces

JEANETTE'S TOP 10 LIST FOR MOTIVATION AND INSPIRATION

1. Going to church on Sunday or Bible study during the week.
2. Music: A great playlist with my favorite songs.
3. Time with family and friends—having fun, talking on the phone, or e-mailing.
4. Reading self-help books: the most memorable for me include *The Seat of the Soul* by Gary Zukav; *Creating Affluence* and *The Seven Spiritual Laws of Success* by Deepak Chopra; *The Four Agreements* by Don Miguel Ruiz; and *Battlefield of the Mind* by Joyce Meyer.
5. Walking, hiking, and playing with my dogs.
6. Being close to nature: the ocean, trees, birds, flowers, animals.
7. Taking a yoga or dance class.
8. Reading quotes or prayers such as the Serenity Prayer: "God grant me the serenity to accept the things I cannot change; the courage to change the things I can; and the wisdom to know the difference."
9. Contemplating passages from the Bible. Among my favorites: "Do nothing from selfishness or empty conceit, but with humility of mind let each of you regard one another as more important than himself; do not merely look out for your own personal interests, but also for the interests of others." Philippians 2:3–4.
10. Reading to discover new ideas and get information I can use in my own life and teaching.

TODAY'S WORKOUT

CARDIO BURN; STRETCH-IT-OUT
Refer to Chapter 22 for your specific cardio workout and correct form.

BREAKING THE HABIT OF LATE-NIGHT SNACKING

Angela is a wife, mother of two, and career woman who works full time. After having her second child she started changing her lifestyle. She only lost ten pounds, but look at the amazing change in her body. She lost 10% body fat and completely reshaped her body. Don't get hung up on the scale!

"Late-night eating is the major unhealthy habit that I've been able to break," confessed Angela. "It used to be that when seven o'clock rolled around and my favorite TV shows started, I associated this time with snacking—on potato chips, chocolate peanut M&M's, or buttered popcorn. Now I only watch television once a week, as I am busy exercising the other days, and I rarely eat after six o'clock. I have low-fat popcorn and reduced-sugar hot chocolate as my treats when I need them!"

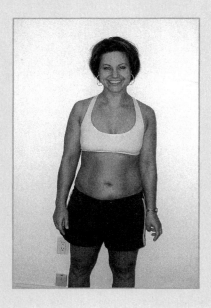 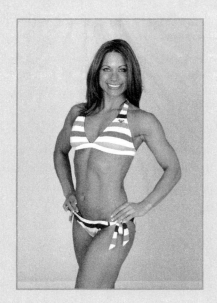

GETTING STARTED

Before you take the first step of today's workout, tell a friend or someone in your family that you are starting a new exercise program, and that today is the first day. Let them know that you are going to be working out six out of seven days from now on, and that you would love company whenever they feel like joining you.

The great thing about a cardio workout is that you don't need a single piece of equipment—and you don't even have to leave your house if you don't want to, although I think it's best to get out into the world and really enjoy various environments. I've designed these workouts so that you can do them anywhere: on a treadmill, at the gym, outside at the park, on a school track or football field, at the beach, or even around the streets of your neighborhood; just make sure you choose a place that is safe and convenient.

The cardio workout offers twelve levels. Everyone has their own starting point, and I want to make sure that you have room to grow wherever you begin. It's crucial to start at the right level so you don't get injured, or just as bad, get discouraged and quit. How did you score on the Rockport Fitness Walking Test? If you scored low or fair, I recommend starting at Level 1; if you scored average, good, or excellent, start at Level 2 or higher. Remember, when in doubt, start low, complete the workout feeling good, and then move up. This program is about *your* success, and the last thing you want is to push it too hard, hurt yourself, and lose steam.

In a 30-minute power walk/jog you will burn approximately 250 to 350 calories, depending on your level of fitness, your body composition, and your genetics. To eliminate some of the guesswork, I recommend that you use a heart rate monitor during your workouts. Using the monitor will also signal you when you are slacking off so you can pump up the energy and make sure you're getting the most out of your workouts. For reference, use Chapter 22: Cardio Burn and Chapter 23: Stretch-It-Out. And, as I always suggest, consult your health-care provider before beginning any new diet or exercise program.

If you want to turn your body into a fat-burning machine, you need to build your aerobic base through cardiovascular exercise; the more you improve your aerobic base, the more efficient you become at using fat as a source of fuel.

Record your heart rate and workout information in your Cardio Log, located in the back of this book (or print out the form available at www.thehollywoodtrainer.com). It is important for you to keep a record of what you accomplish.

Daily Reflection

In the Mental/Physical/Spiritual section of your journal write about the positive, rewarding aspects of your day as well as the challenges—and how you can overcome them. Take note of the things that bring you special joy. Journaling will give you an outlet to release negative experiences and reinforce positive ones. It is a valuable tool when you use it. I know how difficult it can be to remember to write in your journal, so I will ask you various questions at the end of each day to help remind you to get started. You have free range to write whatever makes you feel good, so explore your emotions and release them with your pen and paper.

Music is an excellent source of motivation to help push you through your workouts. Music can help:

- motivate you to complete the workout.
- give you a boost of energy, especially when one of your favorite songs is playing.
- keep you rockin' to increase your intensity and burn more calories.
- increase your enjoyment so you are more consistent with your training.
- inspire you to do your best.

For the first week of the program, I have provided you with seven timeless playlists, choosing music from *Billboard* Top 40, hip-hop, old school, R & B, rock, pop, gospel, and sounds of nature.

Try this *Billboard* Top 40 playlist for today's workout and I guarantee that you will breeze through it.

"Don't Phunk with My Heart" by the Black Eyed Peas
"Lose Control" by Missy Elliott
"Get Right" (Louis Vega Club Mix) by Jennifer Lopez
"Grillz" by Nelly featuring Paul Wall, Ali and Gipp
"Heard 'Em Say" by Kanye West featuring Adam Levine
"Lose My Breath" (Peter Rauhofer's Breathless mix) by Destiny's Child
"We Belong Together" (Remix) by Mariah Carey featuring Jadakiss and Styles P.
"Slow Jamz" (Collipark Remix) by Twista
"Don't Cha" (Remix) by Pussycat Dolls
"Holla Back Girl" by Gwen Stefani
"Touch It" by Busta Rhymes

For new playlists with up-to-the-minute hottest music, visit www.thehollywoodtrainer.com

1. What two qualities do I already possess that will help me adopt new healthy habits?
2. What's one positive characteristic I have that friends and family have brought to my attention? How can I use this characteristic to help myself in other challenges?
3. What was the biggest challenge of the day?
4. What can I do to overcome this challenge for tomorrow?
5. How do I feel after completing my first day?

DAY 2

Courage is saying "Maybe what I'm doing isn't working; maybe I should try something else."
—*Anna Lappé*

Sometimes it takes a lot to recognize the need for change in your life—and even more to do something about it. Changing your habits and your daily behavior is hard, but you *can* do it!

> *Today's Affirmation*
> I realize that change is necessary to create new outcomes, and accept
> that only through change can I improve the quality of my life.
> I am courageous and committed to making new choices.

CHANGING YOUR WORLD

The world is full of things that we can't control, but there are some things we can. If you create an environment that supports your new healthy lifestyle, you are much more likely to achieve your goals. But it all starts with you: today look at how to create an environment that will help you win.

1. Go through your kitchen and get rid of all junk food. It's hard to resist temptation. (And I don't want to hear any excuses about having children in the house who demand unhealthy foods. You should be setting a positive example by making healthy

food choices for yourself *and* your family. You don't want to set your kids up for diet-related health problems later in life.)

2. Stock up on healthy snacks: fresh fruits like blueberries, oranges, grapefruit, apples, melon, or mangoes; healthy nuts such as walnuts or almonds; low-fat yogurt; cut-up vegetables, including carrots, cucumber, or celery; and healthy dips and sauces such as hummus or low-fat cottage cheese. (Refer to the nutrition section and meal plans for healthy recipes.)

3. Instead of meeting friends at the coffee shop or a restaurant, try taking a walk together or going to the gym.

4. When you go to the movies, be prepared: bring your own healthy snack, such as air-popped popcorn, soy nuts, walnuts and dried cranberries, dried fruit, trail mix, or baked chips.

5. Eat a healthy snack or light meal before a party or meeting where you know food will be served. It will help you to resist unhealthy options.

TODAY'S FOOD

THINKING FOODS

Your brain and nervous system need carbohydrates for fuel, which is why we sometimes refer to carbs as "thinking foods." It's very important to eat complex carbohydrates at breakfast and lunch so that you can maintain energy throughout the day and think clearly without being irritable or on edge. The complex-carbohydrate foods in today's menu are oatmeal, yam, and brown-rice cake.

The Menu

* *

Recipes marked with an asterisk (*) can be found in the recipe section, Chapter 17.

BREAKFAST: Oatmeal–Egg White Breakfast Frittata*
SNACK: 1 apple
LUNCH: Grilled Chicken Breasts*/ Garlic Spinach*/ ½ cup baked yam

SNACK: Tomato Cucumber Salad*

SNACK: 1 brown-rice cake with 1 tablespoon soy nut butter and 1 tablespoon all-fruit blueberry jam

DINNER: Albacore Tuna Chopped Salad*

DESSERT: Apple Walnut Dessert*

WATER: Half your body weight in ounces

TODAY'S WORKOUT

CHEST, TRI'S, AND BOOTY (CIRCUIT A); CORE; STRETCH-IT-OUT

For your specific workout and proper form, refer to Chapter 24: Chest, Tri's, and Booty; Chapter 25: Core; and Chapter 23: Stretch-It-Out.

TIME-SAVING AND EFFECTIVE WORKOUT TIPS

Today's workout should take you less than an hour, but be patient because it is your first time going through the exercises. If you are running short on time you can start your day with the Chest, Tri's, and Booty Circuit, then do the Core Workout in the evening before you go to bed. Remember to pay yourself with your time and energy before you pay the rest of the world. Grab your Circuit Training Log to record your weight, repetitions, sets, resting time, and heart rate.

Resistance exercises within the circuits will help you build more active muscle, which will help you burn more calories and more fat, even after you're done exercising. Your goal is to move from one exercise to the next in each circuit *without taking a break*. You should be able to execute each exercise with perfect form and technique before you move to the next level. Even though you are supposed to do the exercises in rapid succession, it is important not to rush through the exercises themselves. Stay focused on the movements you are making and be aware of the body part that you are working. Don't start daydreaming or thinking about the never-ending to-do list ahead of you—feel your muscles as they make every contraction. Quality movement will create top results.

Daily Reflection

On this day, answer the following questions in your journal:

1. What is the one thing in my daily life that I really want to change? What five actions can I take to make that change?
2. What was the biggest challenge of the day?
3. What can I do to overcome this challenge for tomorrow?
4. What was the most rewarding part of my day?

Pump up your workout with today's rock and pop playlist.

"Beautiful Day" by U2

"Because of You" by Kelly Clarkson

"Speed of Sound" by Coldplay

"Under Pressure" by Queen

"Unbelievable" by EMF

"Seven Nation Army" by The White Stripes

"One" by Mary J. Blige featuring U2

"Numb/Encore" (Remix) by Jay-Z and Linkin Park

"Roxanne" by The Police

"Bohemian Rhapsody" by Queen

For new playlists with up-to-the-minute hottest music, visit www.thehollywoodtrainer.com.

DAY 3

The greatest discovery of my generation is that a human being
can alter his life by altering his attitudes of mind.
—*William James*

If you can believe it, you can achieve it. Your mind is powerful and yet difficult to alter. As we get older, we get so stuck in our ways, our opinions, or our preconceived ideas that we often block our own blessings. It is time to get out of your own way, clear all of the negative thoughts and judgments out of your mind, and change your attitude. Be open to a new way of thinking. You have to be your biggest fan and believe in yourself in order to be successful.

> *Today's Affirmation*
> I believe that I can successfully adopt healthy lifestyle habits and
> permanently change my life for the better. I can do it!

CREATING A SELF-FULFILLING PROPHECY

A self-fulfilling prophecy is a prediction you make that becomes true simply by virtue of the fact that you believe it—and keep believing it—until it happens. The person who says "I never win anything" never does win anything. The person who never expects to find a good relationship ends up alone because she's too busy feeling negative. Now is the time to believe in you. There is power in thought and word. I want you to say right now, out loud, "I am going to change my life, my body, my mind, and my soul by adopting healthy habits. I can do it! Watch me flourish, watch me succeed, this is going to happen." I want you to say the words, "I can do it!" at least ten times a day from now on. It may sound too trite, but trust me, if you keep saying it, it will become true.

Next, I want you to write the statement, "I can do it!" on ten sticky notes or small pieces of paper—and feel free to add any encouraging words of your own. Put one of these notes on the fridge door, on the dashboard of your car if you have one, on your nightstand, by your mirror, in your wallet, in your journal, in your Bible or other spiritual book, on the back of your cell phone or PDA, in your top drawer at work, on the front cover of this book, and anywhere else you'll see it. These words of encouragement will remind you throughout the day that you *are* going to reach your goals.

TODAY'S FOOD

FIBER, FIBER, FIBER

Choose carbohydrates that contain fiber; you want to make sure you are getting at least 5 grams per serving and a daily range of 25 to 32 grams for women and 38 to 45 grams for men. Fiber slows the absorption of sugar into the blood, allowing your body to continue burning fat, preventing hypoglycemia (high blood sugar), and reducing your long-term risk of diabetes. Today's menu features whole wheat bread and pita, tomatoes, turkey chili, an orange, and organic baby greens.

The Menu

* *

Recipes marked with an asterisk (*) can be found in the recipe section, Chapter 17.

BREAKFAST: Cheese-y Egg White Omelet*, 1 Chef Ronnda's Turkey Sausage Patty*/1 slice whole wheat bread with 1 tablespoon all-fruit blueberry jam

SNACK: ½ cup organic low-fat/low-sodium cottage cheese with a medium tomato, sliced, seasoned with ground black pepper

LUNCH: Mom's Turkey Vegetable Chili*/half of a 6-inch whole wheat pita

SNACK: 1 orange

SNACK: 8 ounces low-sodium vegetable juice

DINNER: Baked Lemon-Herb Chicken*/Pear–Pine Nut Salad*

DESSERT: Dark Chocolate–Covered Strawberries*

WATER: Half your body weight in ounces

TODAY'S WORKOUT

Cardio Burn; Stretch-It-Out

If Day 1's cardio burn workout was too easy, then go ahead and take it up to the next level. If you were challenged, then repeat the same level and fill in your Cardio Log. Today I want you to focus on your posture while you are power walking or jogging. Roll your shoulders back and down. Imagine there is a string attached to the crown of your head, pulling your neck and back into alignment. Pull your navel toward your spine and feel the abdominals in your core contract. Try to keep your core muscles contracted throughout the workout.

OXYGEN TO BURN FAT

Your body needs oxygen to burn fat—it's that simple. To increase oxygen consumption during a cardio workout, try inhaling and then exhaling for four strides each time. Once you master

BODY AFTER BABY

Traci Mendez gained 60 pounds during her pregnancy and, like most new moms, was left feeling depressed about her body.

"After I had my son, I was really unhappy with my size and shape," she remembers. "I wouldn't let anyone photograph me because I didn't want a reminder of what I looked like. It only took a few months for me to realize that I would still be a good mom if I took some time out to take care of myself. I always wanted to be there for my family but, like many first-time moms, put my own health and personal needs at the bottom of the list. I had to get back the energetic, happy Traci who loved fashion, style, and dressing up, so I started working out four to five times a week and continued eating healthy. I have lost 66 pounds since my pregnancy, and I have gone from a size 14 to a size 7/8! I am excited again to hit the fashion racks, and my spirit is in a positive place. I know I have to be happy and healthy to set a positive example for my son!"

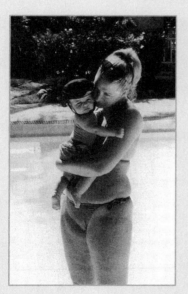 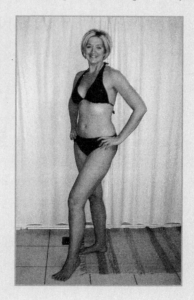

that level, try inhaling for five or six strides and exhaling for the same. Then follow the Stretch-It-Out workout in Chapter 23 (or in *The Hollywood Trainer Weight-Loss Plan Workout* DVD) to feel the benefits of a deep flexibility workout. Remember, this is the day you are required to hold the stretches for 1 to 3 minutes each so that you improve flexibility, release tension, and lengthen muscles.

Pump up your workout with today's hip-hop and R & B playlist.

"My Humps" by the Black Eyed Peas

"On & On" by Missy Elliott

"Get Up" by Ciara

"Heartburn" by Alicia Keys

"(When You Gonna) Give It Up to Me" by Sean Paul featuring Keyshia Cole

"Lighters Up" by Lil' Kim

"Shake It Off" by Mariah Carey

"99 Problems" by Jay-Z

"Hate It or Love It" by Mary J. Blige and The Game

"Ring the Alarm" by Beyoncé

"Make It Clap" by Busta Rhymes featuring Sean Paul

For new playlists with up-to-the-minute hottest music, visit www.thehollywoodtrainer.com.

Daily Reflection

On this day, answer the following questions in your journal:

1. What was the most rewarding part of my day?
2. What are two thoughts or preconceived judgments that other people have made about me? How will I cope with other people judging me?
3. How can I alter my mind to believe in myself, especially in the most challenging times?
4. How do I feel after Day 3?

DAY 4

No people who are ignorant can ever be free.
—*Thomas Jefferson*

Making informed decisions about the food you eat is key to good health. By educating yourself, you can reduce your risk of a number of diseases and conditions, including diabetes, heart disease, hypertension, obesity, atherosclerosis, depression, dementia, fibroids, and even cancer. Knowledge is power!

> *Today's Affirmation*
> If I educate myself about the food I consume on a daily basis, I can take control of my body and ensure that I will make the right choices for a healthy lifestyle.

TODAY'S FOOD

OMEGA-3 FATTY ACIDS

More than 90 percent of Americans are deficient in omega-3 fatty acids, which are an essential fat the body must get from food or in supplement form. On today's menu, your sources of omega-3 fatty acids are flaxseed oil and trout. Omega-3s are very sensitive and are easily destroyed by exposure to oxygen, heat, and light. To be sure you are getting your daily dose, take a fish oil supplement, a tablespoonful of cod liver oil, or 2 ounces of ground flaxseeds. It is important to note that results from a study of 47,000 men published in the *American Journal of Clinical Nutrition* (July 2004; 80(1): 204–216) found that ALA (a type of omega-3 fatty acid found in flaxseeds and other plants) stimulates the growth of prostate tumors in men. This does not mean men ought not consume ALA at all, but it should not be used as a replacement for fish oil supplements. Scientists also found that fish oils (which contain omega-3s EPA and DHA) could reduce the risk of total and advanced prostate cancer. Now it is clear that only a very small percentage of the omega-3s in flaxseed is converted to EPA and DHA. It is actually EPA and DHA that do the heavy lifting for cancer prevention, not ALA. Don't forget all of the amazing fat-burning and health benefits of omega-3 fatty acids. (See Chapter 14, Fat.)

The Menu

Recipes marked with an asterisk (*) can be found in the recipe section, Chapter 17.

BREAKFAST: Whole Wheat Breakfast Burrito*
SNACK: ½ of a medium cantaloupe
LUNCH: Quick-and-Easy Turkey Tomato Penne*/Broccoli Parmesan*
SNACK: 2 large celery stalks with 2 tablespoons organic low-fat cream cheese
SNACK: 1 apple and 1 string organic low-fat cheese
DINNER: Baked Romano Wild Trout*/Garlic Spinach*/Baked Butternut Squash*
DESSERT: ½ cup lemon sorbet with ½ cup fresh berries
WATER: Half your body weight in ounces

TODAY'S WORKOUT

BACK, BI'S, AND THIGHS (CIRCUIT B); CORE; STRETCH-IT-OUT

You can do today's workout by following the guidelines in Part 5 or from *The Hollywood Trainer Weight-Loss Plan Workout* DVD.

I am sure by now you are really feeling muscles that you haven't felt in years. This is great because it means you are right on track to reshaping your body.

Resistance training will help strengthen tendons, ligaments, and bones, which make up your joints; strengthening joints will in turn help reduce the risk of injury from the repetitive motion of cardiovascular activity. If your body is strong, you'll get more out of your workouts, and will see results faster.

Today's workout introduces you to a new circuit, but the same theory applies as before. Keep your body moving between exercises, but be sure to complete each exercise thoroughly and in good form. Focus on the contractions of your muscles, and always remember that quality movement creates top results.

Don't forget to fill out the Circuit Training Log to track your progress throughout the workout.

FLATTEN MY STOMACH!

Liz Scott owns and operates her own thriving company, Organizational Solutions, Inc., in Burlington, Ontario, Canada. She's your classic working mom, who's always on the go with rarely a moment for herself. Liz has an ectomorph body type (long, lean, model-like) and never had weight problems until she reached her forties. Suddenly she noticed her waistline expanding and her clothes getting tighter.

"I started working out in the hopes of bringing back my slender waistline," she says. "Well, it worked! I flattened my stomach and lost 18 pounds and 8 inches. I was able to work out five to six days a week by keeping Jeanette's DVD with me when I was traveling. It's easy to make excuses when you work full time and run a household. I realized that you just *have* to take the time for yourself, because if you don't then you will fall deeper into the unhealthy hole."

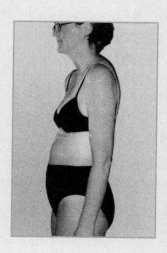

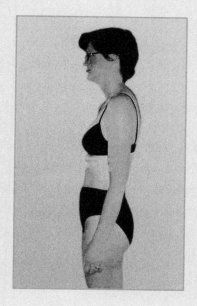

Pump up your workout with today's old-school and disco playlist.

"Give It to Me, Baby" by Rick James
"Let's Groove Tonight" by Earth, Wind & Fire
"Shake Your Booty" by KC and the Sunshine Band
"Outstanding" by the Gap Band
"We Are Family" by Sister Sledge
"Lady Marmalade" by Patti LaBelle
"Best of My Love" by the Emotions
"Le Freak" by Chic
"Ring My Bell" by Anita Ward
"Good Times" by Chic

For new playlists with up-to-the-minute hottest music, visit www.thehollywoodtrainer.com.

Daily Reflection

On this day, answer the following questions in your journal:

1. What are one or two specific things I have learned about health and fitness that I can carry forward on my journey?
2. What was the most rewarding part of the day?
3. What was the most challenging part of the day?
4. What can I do to overcome this challenge?
5. How do I feel after Day 4?

DAY 5

One important key to success is self-confidence.
An important key to self-confidence is preparation.

—*Arthur Ashe*

We live in a world that prizes convenience above almost all else. When it comes to food, however, convenience and good nutrition don't always go hand in hand. In order to make it easier to eat healthy, start thinking more like our grandparents did: buy fresh groceries once a week, and prepare healthy breakfasts and dinners, and wholesome brown-bag lunches. Those of you who work late will have to bring dinner as well—no pizza or Chinese takeout at the office. The best way to be successful with your eating is to accept that you have to plan ahead; you don't want to be at the mercy of the fast-food restaurants, cafeterias, or convenience-food manufacturers, who care far more about shelf life and the bottom line than they do about your health. Prepare ahead and you'll succeed!

> *Today's Affirmation*
> I will prepare by planning my workouts, rest, and meals, and
> I will succeed at achieving my health and fitness goals.

TODAY'S FOOD

THINK AHEAD

Prepare tomorrow's lunch and snacks while you are fixing tonight's dinner. Or use the leftovers from dinner for tomorrow's snacks and lunch. You can also cook and freeze such items as vegetarian or turkey chili or turkey meat loaf in bulk, then thaw and reheat when you need them. Clean and cut veggies and store in water in the fridge so that they are fresh and ready to eat when you want a snack.

The Menu

. . . .

The recipes marked with an asterisk (*) can be found in the recipe section, Chapter 17.

BREAKFAST: Smoked Salmon Bagel with a "Schmear"*
SNACK: 8 ounces low-sodium tomato juice
LUNCH: Turkey Pita Sandwich* (with hummus)
SNACK: ½ of a medium cantaloupe
SNACK: 6 ounces low-fat yogurt
DINNER: Curried Chicken Salad*
DESSERT: ½ cup applesauce
WATER: Half your body weight in ounces

TODAY'S WORKOUT

CHEST, TRI'S, AND BOOTY (CIRCUIT A); STRETCH-IT-OUT

Don't forget to time yourself to see how long it takes you to do Circuit A from start to finish. It's not a race; you should still be paying attention to every muscle contraction during every exercise, and completing every motion with the proper form. Each set has a number of repetitions, or it may be a series of extended holds, such as the plank or the chair pose. Make a note of your time in your journal.

As you finish up with the total body stretches, focus on your breath: once you are in the stretch, concentrate on taking long breaths in and out, inhaling for 4 seconds and exhaling for the same, repeating this 4 times—feel the stretch.

OVERLOAD YOUR MUSCLES

You have to really make your muscles work to create a change in your muscle tone and definition. In order to do that, use enough weight when you are performing the circuit-training exercises. If you can push or pull the weight three or four more times above the prescribed number of reps, then you are probably not using a heavy enough weight. It is important that you use the maximum amount of weight that you can lift with good form. As a beginner you should start with light weights to make sure you have good form and technique; as soon as you're comfortable at the beginner's level you can reevaluate your weight load. You always want to give your muscles as much as they can take—that way you know they're changing and growing.

PLANNING FOR SUCCESS

Like many women today, Marsha does it all: cooks, cleans, works full time as a teacher, and, with her husband, raises their three children. She was challenged when figuring out how to fit exercise into her busy day. It didn't take long for Marsha to be convinced that since she is the glue that holds her family together, *her* health is of utmost importance. As soon as she started the program the entire family enjoyed benefits of a healthier lifestyle. "I was successful because I stuck to a plan and a schedule," Marsha says. "I knew exactly what meals I was preparing every night, and I picked up the groceries on the way home from work for dinner. Being prepared was one of the keys to my success. I have lost 22 pounds and 12 inches!"

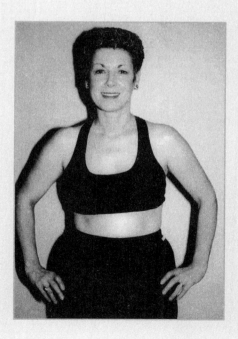 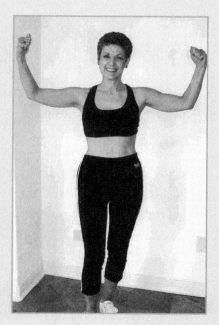

Pump up your workout with today's country music playlist.

"That Don't Impress Me Much" by Shania Twain

"The Lucky One" by Faith Hill

"Something Like That" by Tim McGraw

"Something's Gotta Give" by LeAnn Rimes

"Redneck Woman" by Gretchen Wilson

"There's Your Trouble" by Dixie Chicks

"Boot Scootin' Boogie" by Brooks & Dunn

"Man! I Feel Like a Woman!" by Shania Twain

"Days Go By" by Keith Urban

"How Do You Like Me Now?!" by Toby Keith

"Ashes by Now" by Lee Ann Womack

For new playlists with up-to-the-minute hottest music, visit www.thehollywoodtrainer.com.

Daily Reflection

On this day, answer the following questions in your journal:

1. What was the most rewarding part of the day?
2. What can I prepare in advance to help me fit in workouts and eat healthy?
3. What was the most challenging part of today's program?
4. What can I do to overcome this challenge?
5. How do I feel after Day 5?

DAY 6

A strong positive mental attitude will create more miracles than any wonder drug.
—Patricia Neal

We've all heard the expression about the glass that's either half empty or half full. And you probably know that if you see the glass as half empty—when you focus your energies on what's missing—*you're* missing out on the opportunity to ignite your heart and soul with positive energy. A pessimistic attitude blocks the blessings you deserve. Your approach to every situation in life has a major effect on its outcome, as well as on your mental and spiritual health. If you approach a situation with anger, resignation, or negativity, then you are not going to get a positive outcome. By the same token if you have an open mind and a compassionate heart, you will get the same in return. Today, make a special effort: for every situation that arises I want you to be understanding, loving, and patient. No matter what comes up, react in a caring, proactive way, with a smile on your face and love in your heart. A positive attitude is the best antidepressant on the market—it's also free and doesn't have any bad side effects. Plus, it's contagious and will affect everyone around you. Try it out for a day and I guarantee you'll feel great.

> *Today's Affirmation*
> I will approach every situation with a smile and a positive attitude!

TODAY'S FOOD

READ FOOD LABELS AND INGREDIENTS LISTS

When you go grocery shopping it's important to read food labels thoroughly; a lot of nasty chemicals, additives, and preservatives can be hidden in the ingredients list. At first glance, the nutritional information on a packaged product will look fine—no trans fats or only three grams of sugar. However, the chemicals hiding in the ingredients list can still do your body harm. To give you an idea of what I'm talking about, let's take a look at the contents of three different kinds of bread, all of which sound pretty healthy: organic whole wheat, organic sprouted grain, and light whole wheat.

Whole Foods Organic 100% Whole Wheat Bread (1 slice, 110 calories): whole wheat flour, water, canola oil, vital wheat gluten, sea salt, yeast, cultured wheat flour, enzymes (wheat flour, enzymes, ascorbic acid).

Food for Life Organic Sprouted Grain Bread Ezekiel 4:9 Low-Sodium (1 slice, 80 calories): organic sprouted wheat, organic sprouted barley, organic sprouted millet, organic malted barley, organic sprouted lentils, organic sprouted soybeans, organic sprouted spelt, filtered water, fresh yeast.

Oroweat 100% Whole Wheat Light Bread (2 slices, 80 calories): water, whole wheat flour, wheat gluten, oat fiber, soy fiber, molasses, fructose, cracked wheat, yeast, salt, wheat bran, nonfat milk, barley, wheat fiber, brown sugar, dextrose, natural flavor, calcium propionate (preservative), rye malt, soybean oil, sodium stearoyl lactylate, mono and diglycerides, guar gum, xanthan gum, ethoxylated mono and diglycerides, monocalcium phosphate, soy lecithin, carrageenan gum, propylene glycol, caramel color, ascorbic acid.

Each of these organic bread has only have nine ingredients compared with the thirty-plus ingredients that are in the conventional/nonorganic whole wheat light bread. Think about it: can it really be necessary to add more than twenty extra ingredients to *bread*? The fact is, these ingredients are only there to keep expenses for raw materials as low as possible, and to extend shelf life and increase profits. Of the three breads examined here, I would definitely pick the Food for Life organic sprouted grain bread or the Whole Foods Organic 100% Whole Wheat—the least expensive and the healthiest! I also understand all of the ingredients and know that they have not undergone refinement or processing but are left for me to consume as God intended.

The Menu

. . . .

Recipes marked with an asterisk (*) can be found in the recipe section, Chapter 17.

BREAKFAST: Fruit Platter with Cottage Cheese*
SNACK: 14 walnuts mixed with 2 tablespoons dried cranberries

LUNCH: Tofu Vegetable Stir-fry*/½ cup cooked brown rice

SNACK: 1 cup raw baby carrots/2 large celery stalks/4 tablespoons hummus dip

SNACK: 1 apple/1 string organic low-fat cheese

DINNER: Halibut with Mango Salsa*/Roasted Asparagus*

DESSERT: 6 ounces Greek yogurt and ½ cup fresh berries garnished with 3 tablespoons low-fat granola

WATER: Half your body weight in ounces

COMMITMENT, CONSISTENCY, AND MOM'S SUNDAY BRUNCH

Myron's goal was weight loss, and he accomplished his goal by accepting that he had to make changes and then stay committed. Commitment and consistency are absolutely necessary to achieve weight-loss success. "I stick to the workout program and healthy eating all week," says Myron, "but when Sunday comes, I give in to Mom's Sunday brunch. Indulging once a week in some of my favorite foods with friends and family is nurturing to my soul. I realize that moderation is the key and that I can indulge only once a week and then it is back to my healthy lifestyle on Monday. I have lost more than 50 pounds and more than 23 inches from my body by being consistent and staying committed to eating healthy and working out."

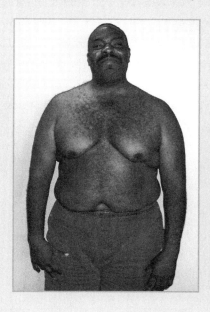
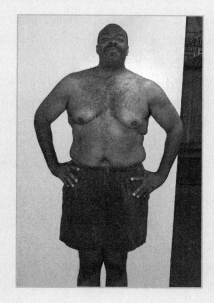

TODAY'S WORKOUT

BACK, BI'S, AND THIGHS (CIRCUIT B); CORE; STRETCH-IT-OUT

Refer to Part 5 or *The Hollywood Trainer Weight-Loss Plan Workout* DVD for specific exercises and correct form.

You've already been through the exercises in Circuit B, so now let's see if you can improve your form. Focus on the muscles that are being recruited in each exercise, and make sure you actually feel the muscle being used. Start executing each exercise with deliberate intention. If you're doing a back row, feel the muscles in your upper back, shoulders, and biceps contracting each time you complete a rep. Research has shown that when you are mentally in tune and engaged with the exercises you are doing, you actually recruit more muscle fibers. Concentrate on perfecting each movement, and watch the improvement in your form and your physique.

DROP SETS

Drop sets are added in Level 2 of both circuits, and they will help you recruit all three muscle fiber types to create more active muscle. The more active muscle you create, the more calories and body fat you will be burning, whether you're working out or watching TV. To perform a drop set, start with the heaviest weight you can lift with good form and do 12 to 15 reps before immediately dropping the weight by 25 to 50 percent to complete 10 to 13 more reps for a total of 25. Doing drop sets will also help you get more definition and tone in your muscles.

Daily Reflection

On this day, answer the following questions in your journal:

1. Have I tried my best to handle every situation today with a smile and a positive attitude?
2. What was the most challenging part of the day and what can I do about it?
3. What was the most rewarding part of the day?
4. How do I feel after Day 6?

Pump up your workout with today's gospel music playlist.

"Heaven" by Mary Mary
"The Blessing of Abraham" by Donald Lawrence
"We Acknowledge You" by Karen Clark Sheard
"Sing!" by Micah Stampley
"Pray" by CeCe Winans
"Victory" by Yolanda Adams
"Looking for You" by Kirk Franklin
"The Real Party (Trevon's Birthday)" by Mary Mary
"No Way" by Tye Tribbett and the Greater Anointing Chant
"We Fall Down but We Get Up" by Donnie McClurkin

For new playlists with up-to-the-minute hottest music, visit www.thehollywoodtrainer.com.

DAY 7

I believe that the very purpose of our life is to seek happiness. That is clear. Whether one believes
in religion or not, whether one believes in this religion or that religion, we all are seeking
something better in life. So, I think, the very motion of our life is toward happiness.

Happiness is not something ready-made. It comes from your own actions.
—*His Holiness the Dalai Lama*

You have so much power in your actions, attitude, and approach. Think about all of the people
you enjoy spending time with—they are usually happy, positive, or generous individuals. No
one wants to spend time with a Debbie Downer. Negative people who spend all of their energy

complaining are toxic. Think before you speak and before you take action. Are you being a Debbie Downer? Your friends, family, and coworkers would much rather see a smile on your face and hear positive, loving words. Your happiness will improve dramatically if you choose to be generous, loving, and happy toward others. The happiness you put out into the universe will come back to you tenfold.

Today's Affirmation
I take full responsibility for my actions. I am responsible for my own happiness.

TODAY'S FOOD

TRANSFORM YOUR FAVORITE MEAL

Take one of your favorite meals and turn it into a healthy alternative by replacing some of the ingredients with lighter substitutes. Two of my favorite foods are pancakes and lasagna, and I've included recipes for healthy versions in today's menu.

The Menu

Recipes marked with an asterisk (*) can be found in the recipe section, Chapter 17.

BREAKFAST: Blueberry and Banana Buckwheat Pancakes*
SNACK: 2 hard-boiled eggs, mashed and seasoned with a dash of salt and ground black pepper
LUNCH: Turkey Lasagna*
SNACK: ½ a Tuna Pita Sandwich*
SNACK: 3 oz. smoked salmon on 5 low-fat whole wheat crackers
DINNER: Turkey Meat Loaf*/Roasted Acorn Squash*/Lemon Green Beans*
DESSERT: California Fruit Salad*
WATER: Half your body weight in ounces

TODAY'S WORKOUT

REST, RELAX, AND REJUVENATE

Today—whether it's the weekend or midweek—would be a good day to think about clearing your thoughts, stilling the mind, and getting into that deeper part of yourself that you've been neglecting. A day of rest can be any day of the week that works with your schedule. Bring all your attention to your soul so you can tap your most powerful and creative aspects and let them out.

Run a nice hot bath, light some candles and incense, and enjoy being still. Let your mind, body, and soul completely unwind. You might book a massage for yourself —you'd be amazed how restorative it can be to take time for a little pampering. You might even be more productive during the rest of the week.

A PLACE TO RELAX

Create a space to relax, meditate, and replenish.

1. Pick a location: in the garden close to nature, in a corner of your bedroom, at a community park or garden, in a special room in your home, or in a corner of your office.
2. Have on hand a symbol that will help you relax: a candle, a cross, a star, a heart, a photo, or a plant.
3. Keep incense or aromatherapy oils in such fragrances as eucalyptus, lavender, jasmine, juniper breeze, or nagchampa to help create a relaxing atmosphere through your sense of smell.
4. Bring a warm blanket that will help your body feel warmth so you can relax.

Use this space to close your eyes and escape from the world. You can focus on a calming breath or visualization to help you relax and be still. You may feel uncomfortable at first, but just 5 or 10 minutes on your most stressful days will help you release negative energy from your body. Try to take some time at least once or twice a week, and you can build up slowly until you are doing it every day. Relaxation is an art—make sure you do it right, and get as much out of it as you can.

Enjoy your leisure time with this relaxation and meditation playlist.

"Only Time" by Enya
Amazon Rainforests by Sounds of Nature
Relaxation and Meditation with Music and Nature by Classical Sounds of Nature
Caribbean Sounds by Sounds of Nature
Bach by Classical Relaxation
Mozart by Classical Relaxation
Relaxation Aboriginal Didgeridoo by African Drums
"Chinese Folk Music/ Thai Chi Ch'uan Way" by Oliver Shanti & Friends

Daily Reflection

On this day, answer the following questions in your journal:

1. What can I do to create a happier environment for my friends and family?
2. Did I really rest on my day off? If not, is it possible to rearrange my schedule so that I can fit in a whole day of real rest, and truly rejuvenate myself for the new week ahead?
3. What was the most rewarding part of my day?
4. What was the most challenging part of my week?
5. What can I do to overcome this challenge?
6. How do I feel after Day 7?
7. How do I feel about my efforts over the past week? Am I doing my best to change my life and make healthier choices for my mind, body, and soul?

DAY 8

Learn from yesterday, live for today, hope for tomorrow. The important thing is not to stop questioning.
—Albert Einstein

There is no such thing as a stupid question. Asking questions and looking for answers is part of the learning process. Learn from the many experiences that you have gone through, but don't let those experiences define you as a person. Live for today with love, happiness, and kindness because you are never promised tomorrow. Move forward with determination to achieve your goals, faith that you will attain them, and confidence that you will succeed.

> *Today's Affirmation*
>
> I will learn from my past experiences and live in the present moment with kindness and compassion. I will look forward with faith and confidence that I will continue to be blessed. I will not be afraid to ask questions because I know that education will empower me.

LEARN FROM THE PAST

Look back and think of two things that you can learn from your first week on the plan that will help you in your second. Make a note of them in your journal.

LIVE FOR THE PRESENT

Your workout time is for you—not your job, not your cell phone, BlackBerry, or anything else. Try to live in the moment physically and mentally. It's easy to get distracted by everything that's going on in your life, but don't cheat yourself of this time; give your mind, body, and soul your undivided attention.

HOPE FOR THE FUTURE

You may have run into challenges during your first week. Guess what: you're human, not perfect, and everyone slips up every once in a while. It's okay. The good news? You have the power to direct the future, and it's a whole lot easier to do so if you face it with a hopeful, positive attitude. As you enter your second week, remember that you have the power to make every situation work in your favor. Stay hopeful. Think of at least one thing coming up in your week ahead that you will need to approach with a positive attitude, and make a note of it in your journal as a daily reminder.

ASK QUESTIONS ALONG THE WAY
The workings of your body and the science of nutrition are complicated topics, and I'm sure there are still areas that seem confusing to you. If you need a refresher course or want further clarification on anything, here are a few things you can try:

1. Reread sections of this book that are still unclear. Sometimes things start making sense as you are doing them, so now that you've started the program it may be easier to connect the dots.
2. Do a little research on the Internet, but always make sure to evaluate your source. There is a list of useful Web sites in the Appendix as well as on my Web site, www.thehollywoodtrainer.com.
3. Ask questions—at your doctor's office, local gym, and health food store. There are experts all around you—learn from them.

TODAY'S FOOD

DAILY PROTEIN INTAKE
Protein is necessary to rebuild active muscle, and active muscle burns fat. You should be consuming approximately 1 gram of protein for each pound of ideal lean body weight. If your goal weight is 140 pounds and 28 percent body fat, then your ideal is 140lbs − (140lbs × 28%) = 100.8 lbs. Therefore, you should be consuming 100.8 grams of protein. Today's major protein selections are eggs, ground turkey, yogurt, and salmon. Make sure that you have a protein at breakfast, lunch, dinner, and sometimes one or two snacks to make sure you get the required amount of this essential nutrient. Your body cannot produce its own protein, so you must get it from your diet, even if you are a vegetarian.

The Menu

· ·

Recipes marked with an asterisk (*) can be found in the recipe section, Chapter 17.

BREAKFAST: Egg White–Turkey Scramble*

SNACK: 8 ounces low-sodium tomato juice

LUNCH: Quick-and-Easy Chicken Caesar Salad*

SNACK: Roasted Acorn Squash*

SNACK: 6 ounces Greek yogurt with ½ cup fresh berries garnished with 3 tablespoons low-fat granola

DINNER: Poached Wild Salmon*/Black Bean and Corn Salad*

DESSERT: 2 Oatmeal Raisin Cookies*

WATER: Half your body weight in ounces

TODAY'S WORKOUT

Cardio Burn; Stretch-It-Out
Refer to Part 5 for specific exercises and proper form.

PROPER FIT FOR YOUR FEET

Pain in your feet and ankles could be due to ill-fitting running shoes. Do you know what kind of foot you have? Are you a flat foot? Do you overpronate? Do you underpronate/supinate? If you experience discomfort in your feet when you are walking, jogging, or running, then make an appointment with a podiatrist or spend some time in a specialty running-shoe store where someone can examine your gait and match your foot with the perfect shoe for you. (See Chapter 21.)

Make sure you fill in your Cardio Log for today's workout. Monitor your heart rate and put in 110 percent.

Daily Reflection

On this day, answer the following questions in your journal:

1. What did I learn from the first week that can help me improve my nutrition plan and workout program?
2. What was the most challenging part of the day?
3. What can I do to overcome this challenge?
4. What was the most rewarding part of the day?

A WOMAN ON A MISSION

Taji is a clinical psychologist who has the kind of mental strength and energy you wish came in a bottle. However, at 205 pounds, she was feeling physically defeated. That's when she made the choice and commitment to turn her life around. When Taji first came to my class, I responded instantly to her positive energy and made it a point to give her some extra motivation.

"I was working the plan," Taji says, "but Jeanette informed me that I wasn't getting enough protein in my diet or enough strength training in my exercise program to protect my connective tissue and joints from overuse injuries. I have now lost 40 pounds and achieved 10 percent body fat and am certain that I will reach my final goal weight of 140."

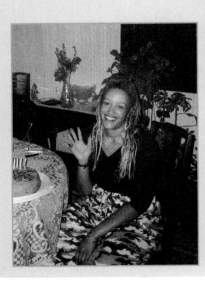
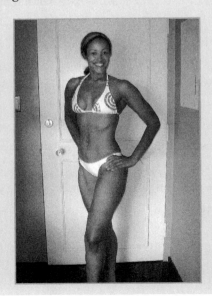

DAY 9

Trust in the Lord with all thine heart, and lean not unto thine own understanding.
In all ways acknowledge Him, and he shall direct thy paths.

—*Proverbs 3:5–6*

A lot of the time people are searching for a clear, black-and-white understanding of a situation. But life is not black-and-white. For every new discovery or claim, there is a contradiction. There is an exception to every rule. Miracles happen and can't be explained. The pieces of your life do not fall into place like a perfect puzzle or timeless painting. Putting your faith in God and maintaining strong morals and values will allow you to let go when you just don't understand. Imagine your morals and values are the strong picture frame but your day-to-day life is the picture within the frame. The frame is strong but the picture will constantly change. Have faith and enjoy each picture because the artist is God.

> *Today's Affirmation*
> I will trust in the Lord and not depend on just my
> own limited understanding. I will acknowledge the Lord in all ways.

FIND A WORKOUT BUDDY

The best workout partner is someone whom you can lean on for support and turn to for inspiration. There are many people who work out on a regular basis who would love to join you on this journey.

- Get involved with a regular cardio class like indoor cycling, walking, step, dance, boxing, or aerobics at the gym or community center. By communicating and introducing yourself to the regular students in the class you can start to create a supportive environment.
- Post a sign at a gym, your workplace, school, or community center for a workout buddy during the time frame that works for you.

- Ask one of your girlfriends or family members and it will also be an opportunity for you to share laughs and time together. Yes, starting a workout program can be funny, even hilarious. I encourage the laughter—it's great for your spirit!

TODAY'S FOOD

ORGANIC BEEF VERSUS CONVENTIONAL BEEF

Red meat that is grass fed and organic is your best bet. Red meat has been given a bad rap in the past twenty years due to the negative side effects that people have had from the "food" that has been fed to cows, everything from cement filler to feces. Conventional cows have also been pumped with steroids and hormones. Meat from healthy cows that get to eat grass and have not been treated with pesticides and herbicides will not leave you with negative side effects. You can find a source for organic beef on the Internet or visit grocers such as Whole Foods, Wild Oats, and Trader Joe's.

The Menu

The recipes marked with an asterisk (*) can be found in the recipe section, Chapter 17.

BREAKFAST: Jeanette's California Sunshine Protein Smoothie*
SNACK: 2 hard-boiled eggs, mashed and seasoned with a dash of salt and ground black pepper
LUNCH: Asian Chicken Stir-fry*
SNACK: 1 cup uncooked broccoli florets/1 cup baby carrots/4 tablespoons hummus dip
SNACK: 1 brown-rice cake with ½ cup low-fat cottage cheese and 2 tomato slices seasoned with a dash of ground black pepper
DINNER: Broiled Sirloin Steak*/Tomato and Red Onion Salad*/Broccoli Parmesan*
DESSERT: Chef Ronnda's Caramelized Apples*
WATER: Half your body weight in ounces

FOOD QUALITY AND FOOD QUANTITY

"When I started working with Jeanette I was on a weight-loss program that focused only on portion size for weight loss," says Amber Dykes. "I soon learned that the quality of food and body fat percentage were just as important as portion sizes and body weight. Now when I eat a meal I'm not only focused on the calories, but also on whether it is made with wholesome ingredients—whole wheat instead of white flour bread, for instance. When I weigh myself at the end of the week, I'm not upset if my weight doesn't go down. I look at other indicators now: Are my clothes getting looser? Is my body fat percentage lower? Am I feeling good about myself? I know that healthy living makes me feel happy and empowered. The physical payoffs are an added plus. I have lost 25 pounds and 18 inches over my body, and I am down four dress sizes."

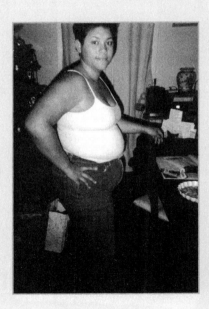 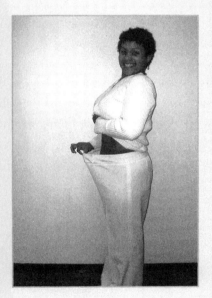

TODAY'S WORKOUT

CHEST, TRI'S, AND BOOTY (CIRCUIT A); CORE; STRETCH-IT-OUT
Refer to Part 5 or follow *The Hollywood Trainer Weight-Loss Plan Workout* DVD for specific exercises and correct form.

CONTINUOUS REPETITIONS

Any set of 15 or 25 repetitions should be continuous. Try not to stop during the middle of a set. If you can keep pushing or pulling the weight with good form and technique, continue until you've completed all of the repetitions in that set. The burning sensation that you feel in your muscle when you're getting close to the end of a set is due to your blood not being able to deliver enough oxygen to your muscles to support their effort. As you improve your level of aerobic fitness, anaerobic fitness, muscular endurance, and muscular strength, your ability to push more weight and more reps will also improve.

Daily Reflection

On this day, answer the following questions in your journal:

1. What is one thing that I try to control that causes me anxiety? Can I turn my concerns over to God and have faith that he will help me find the way?
2. What was the most challenging part of today's program?
3. What can I do to overcome this challenge?
4. What was the most rewarding part of my day?

DAY 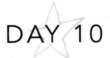 10

One moment of patience may ward off great disaster.
One moment of impatience may ruin a whole life.
—*Chinese proverb*

Millions of people have bought into advertisers' claims that this or that magic pill will make you drop so much weight in so little time. And countless thousands have suffered the bad side effects, from headaches and tremors to nausea and upset stomach or even heart attack or stroke. How does this happen? Whether diet pills are "natural" or not, they all contain drugs that are not naturally found in your body: caffeine, white willow bark, ma huang (a form of ephedra), and hoodia are all things that occur naturally on earth but are still foreign to our bodies. And you will experience a side effect as your body tries to get rid of the unwelcome substance. So the next time you're tempted to reach for a quick-fix solution, stop and think. Be patient, and be smart. Educate yourself. Remember, if you want to lose weight and keep it off for good, you have to create habits that you can maintain for years. Can you take a diet pill for the rest of your life? Obviously not. On the other hand, can you work out and eat healthy for the rest of your life? Yes, you can.

> *Today's Affirmation*
> I will be patient during this process of creating new healthy
> habits and reaching my new lifestyle goals.

TODAY'S FOOD

ENVIRONMENTAL POLLUTANTS

There's a Chinese proverb that says "Each generation will reap what the former generation has sown." Do your part to protect our world by living an environmentally friendly life. Our children are going to suffer from the damage we do to the planet today. The toxins that we've put into the environment—herbicides, pesticides, gas exhaust, and other pollutants—have a direct effect on our food and water supply and, in turn, on our health.

Menu

Recipes marked with an asterisk (*) can be found in the recipe section, Chapter 17.

BREAKFAST: Veggie–Egg White Frittata*/Chef Ronnda's Turkey Sausage Patties*
SNACK: 8 ounces low-sodium tomato juice
LUNCH: Tuna Pita Sandwich*
SNACK: Asian Chicken–Cabbage Salad*

SNACK: 1 brown-rice cake with 3 tomato slices and 2 teaspoons mustard
DINNER: Grilled Chicken Breasts*/Grilled Mixed Vegetables*
DESSERT: Blueberry Mini Cakes*
WATER: Half your body weight in ounces

TODAY'S WORKOUT

Cardio Burn; Stretch-It-Out
Refer to Part 5 for specific cardio levels. Today is flexibility stretching, so you have to hold each stretch for 1 to 3 minutes.

REVIEW STRIDE LENGTH

Remember to turn up the heat and pump your arms while you walk or run. Every time you walk, jog, run, or sprint, focus on engaging your core muscles and creating the largest stride possible while pumping with the opposite arm. Roll your shoulders down and back, take nice long breaths, pull your navel to your spine, and take long strides while pumping the opposite arm, rotating and engaging your core muscles to ignite a fire of intention. You are walking/jogging/running with a purpose. Put in 100 percent and you will feel great. Make each step and pump of the arms count. Pumping your arms will also help you burn more calories and improve the muscular endurance in your upper body.

Daily Reflection

On this day, answer the following questions in your journal:

1. What aspects of my life would benefit from my being more patient?
2. What was the most rewarding part of the day?
3. How do I feel after Day 10?

ANTIAGING! SIXTY-FOUR GOING ON THIRTYSOMETHING

Ms. Charley Johnson runs Charley's Body Factory, a studio in St. Louis where she teaches classes to children as young as four and adults as wise as seventy. At sixty-four years young, Charley moves like a twenty-year-old and is living proof that antiaging is a benefit of a healthy lifestyle. "Healthy living is a way of life that you are never too old to begin," she claims. "I believe I am what I eat—healthy grains, oats, beans, green and leafy vegetables, fruit and fiber. I surround myself with people who are positive and spiritual because I know they have an effect on my life. I drink eight glasses of water a day, exercise at least twelve hours a week, and always try to keep moving. I do not allow problems to take over my life. My family members—especially my grandchildren—are very important to me, and I can keep up with all of them. I love what I do, and I do what I love: exercise and dance. I just celebrated forty-five years of marriage and I love life! Jeanette Jenkins has given me so much more inspiration. I have changed my weekly routine and I am doing even more."

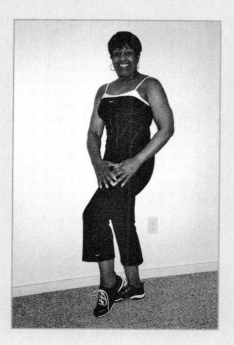

DAY 11

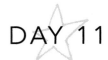

Your time is limited, so don't waste it living someone else's life. Don't be trapped by dogma—which is living with the results of other people's thinking. Don't let the noise of others' opinions drown out your own inner voice. And most important, have the courage to follow your heart and intuition. They somehow already know what you truly want to become. Everything else is secondary.

—*Steve Jobs*

You can define who you are, but you have to believe it to make it true! Your parents, other relatives, friends, colleagues, acquaintances, and society love to define who you are; people will try to characterize you by your hair color, age, gender, occupation, or education. It's important to realize that you must not let anyone else's opinion limit your potential. As long as you are living and breathing, you have to believe with all your heart that anything is possible. You are the only one who has the power to define yourself. Don't accept the limits other people try to put on you.

> • • • *Today's Affirmation* • • •
> I will live my own life and not be defined by the opinions of others. I will follow my heart and trust my own intuition to achieve the life I most want.

TODAY'S FOOD

DAILY REQUIREMENTS OF WATER

Never underestimate the importance of getting enough water. Not only does water make up 60 to 70 percent of your body weight, but water is also needed at the site of the muscle cell to burn fat. When you don't drink enough water, you make it more difficult for your body to function properly. Dr. Fereydoon Batmanghelidj, author of several books related to the body's need for water, has researched the effects of dehydration for more than twenty years and recommends that you drink half of your body weight in ounces of water daily. So if you weigh 180 pounds, then you should probably drink 90 ounces of water a day but the amount you need is going to depend on your body size and activity level.

The Menu

Recipes marked with an asterisk (*) can be found in the recipe section, Chapter 17.

BREAKFAST: Chef Stephanie's Frittata*
SNACK: 1 orange
LUNCH: Chicken Tomato Avocado Pita*
SNACK: Mixed Greens Salad*
SNACK: ½ cup cottage cheese and 5 low-fat whole wheat crackers

DINNER: Turkey Meat Loaf*/Tomato Cucumber Salad*
DESSERT: Apple Crisp*
WATER: Half your body weight in ounces

TODAY'S WORKOUT

BACK, BI'S, AND THIGHS (CIRCUIT B); CORE; STRETCH-IT-OUT
Refer to Part 5 for specific exercises and correct form. Today's stretches are completed during the warm-up and cooldown.

SCHEDULE YOUR WORKOUTS

Try to schedule your workouts for first thing in the morning. We all live busy lives, and sometimes it is difficult to get a workout in the middle of the day, when there are so many things that have to get done. Give your first waking moments of every day to yourself! Starting your day with an energy boost will help you keep a positive attitude and will help keep you more mindful of eating healthy, because you started your day in touch with your body.

Daily Reflection

On this day, answer the following questions in your journal:

1. What are two instances when I let someone's opinion stop me from following my heart?
2. In the future what will I say and do to make sure I follow my heart, dreams, and intuition instead of someone else's opinion?

CHOOSING TO DEFINE HERSELF

Camille is someone who truly hasn't let other people define her life but has taken a journey of renewal that is as much mental and spiritual as it is physical.

"When I was fourteen my seventh-grade teacher and school guidance counselor jointly diagnosed me with a learning disability and told me I had to leave my friends to go into a class with a special teacher," recalls Camille. "This special class kept me from getting the appropriate credentials to enroll in a regular high school, which also prevented me from being able to apply to a regular college. I completed the educational courses required for trade school and mastered the trade of sewing. However, I knew this was not satisfactory for me, so I pushed to enroll at the high school my younger brother and sister were attending. I did continue to college and completed a degree in fashion and merchandising. But after several years, I realized another passion and I began taking flying lessons. I went back to school to get an aviation degree and become a pilot. If I had accepted the diagnosis of my teachers, I never would have become a pilot!"

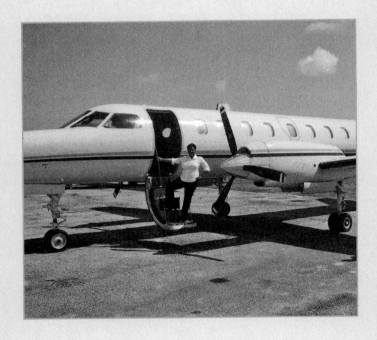

3. What have I done today that makes me feel proud?

4. What changes are occurring in the way I approach eating and working out?

DAY 12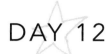

Jealousy . . . is a mental cancer.

—*B. C. Forbes, founder* Forbes *magazine*

Jealousy is an emotion that will destroy your positive light if you let it. Everyone is capable of feeling jealous, but it can become unhealthy for your mind and toxic for your life if you do not reverse the negative feelings and anger that often accompany it. Instead of letting jealousy get the better of you, use the feeling as an opportunity to examine yourself. Why are you having these negative feelings? Are you where you would like to be in your own life? What can you do to achieve your goals? As an exercise to reduce jealousy, congratulate people around you who achieve success and be happy for them, just as you would like them to be happy for you. If you have a generous spirit the universe will be generous with you in return.

> *Today's Affirmation*
> I will use feelings of jealousy as an opportunity to examine where
> I would like to be and what efforts I need to make to achieve my goals.

TODAY'S FOOD

HEALTHY FATS

Healthy and essential fats will give you sustained energy and a satisfied feeling of being full. Essential fats help your body burn fat. Today's healthy fats are in the following food items: egg yolks (choose free-range and enriched in omega-3s), soy nut butter, trout, walnuts, and almonds. Eggs become enriched in omega-3 fatty acids when the chickens are fed flaxseeds. (Review Chapter 14 for more about fats.)

The Menu

* *

Recipes marked with an asterisk (*) can be found in the recipe section, Chapter 17.

BREAKFAST: Cinnamon Berry French Toast*/Chef Ronnda's Turkey Sausage Patties*
SNACK: 2 hard-boiled eggs, mashed and seasoned with a dash of salt and ground pepper
LUNCH: Soft Turkey Taco*
SNACK: 6 ounces Greek yogurt with ½ cup fresh berries garnished with 3 tablespoons, low-fat granola
SNACK: 1 brown-rice cake with 1 tablespoon soy nut butter and ½ tablespoon all-fruit blueberry jam
DINNER: Baked Trout*/Roasted Brussels Sprouts*/Curried Sweet Potato*
DESSERT: Chef Ronnda's Almond Ricotta Cheesecake*
WATER: Half your body weight in ounces

TODAY'S WORKOUT

CHEST, TRI'S, AND BOOTY (CIRCUIT A); STRETCH-IT-OUT
Refer to Part 5 for specific exercises and correct form. Don't forget to end today's workout with the total body stretches.

ANTIDEPRESSANTS VERSUS NATURAL ENDORPHINS

For the millions of people taking antidepressants, I have a natural alternative—and I am not talking about some herb or root. Working out every day is an excellent, healthy, drug-free way to lift your spirits and put you in a great mood, because physical exercise releases endorphins, the "happy hormones," into the bloodstream during and after a workout.

FOOD DRAMA

Brely finds joy in adding music and friends to her workouts but, in her words, "the food thing was always drama.

"I find that a lot of people have problems adopting healthy eating because they live busy lifestyles and they just eat on the run," Brely says. "If you wait until you are hungry to choose something healthy to eat your options are limited. Let's face it, if it doesn't taste good then it is not going to be satisfying and you are still going to feel like you want something else to eat. Sometimes I use a food delivery service because I know I am too busy to prepare my meals, and sometimes I will go grocery shopping and prepare my meals in advance. By planning and preparing dishes ahead, I am satisfied with my meals, I feel great, and I am able to keep the weight off. I have lost 36 pounds and four dress sizes by avoiding the food drama."

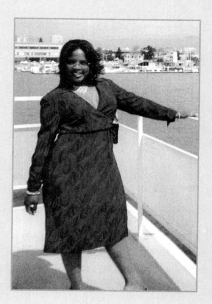 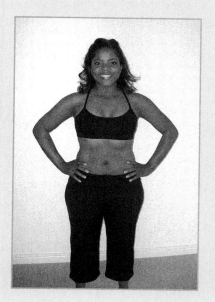

It's time to check your Circuit Training Log to see if you've reduced the time it takes you to do the Chest, Tri's, and Booty (Circuit A) from beginning to end, completing two sets of each circuit with good form and technique. If your time has improved from a week ago, congratulations. Consider taking it to the next level. If your time is the same and you still feel challenged by your current level, then continue to focus on your form. You will create a change in your body as long as your muscles are being challenged.

Remember to schedule your workouts into your daily planner for next week.

Daily Reflection

On this day, answer the following questions in your journal:

1. Do I ever have feelings of jealousy? If so, when and why?
2. What can I do to defeat these negative emotions?
3. What are two or three things that I like about myself?
4. What was the most rewarding part of the day?
5. What have I done today that I'm proud of?
6. How do I feel after Day 12?

DAY 13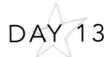

> When one door of happiness closes, another opens; but often we look so long at the
> closed door that we do not see the one which has been opened for us.
> —*Helen Keller*

People often waste energy focusing on past incidents that cannot be changed. The best we can do is to learn what we can from the past and move on with a positive attitude. Whether it's the end of a relationship or the end of a job, we have a tendency to dwell on endings. When we waste energy, especially negative energy complaining about our circumstances, we often block the blessings that are right in front of us.

Today's Affirmation
When I feel that one door is closed to me, I will move on
in search of other positive things that life has in store.

TODAY'S FOOD

PROCESSED FOODS

Processed foods such as white bread, white rice, white pasta, cookies, cakes, muffins, cereals, doughnuts, chips, or pastries are made with such highly refined carbohydrates that your body recognizes them as sugar. These items may list zero grams of sugar on the nutritional information label, but you must look at the fiber content as well. If there is little or no fiber in the food, then this processed food item is going to be absorbed quickly into your bloodstream and raise your blood sugar level, which will cause your body to hold on to its body fat. One of the keys to burning your own body fat is to keep your blood sugar level down.

The Menu

Recipes marked with an asterisk (*) can be found in the recipe section, Chapter 17.

BREAKFAST: Greek Yogurt Crunch*
SNACK: 2 hard-boiled eggs, mashed with a dash of salt and ground black pepper
LUNCH: Salmon Salad Sandwich*
SNACK: One 6-inch whole wheat pita bread stuffed with 4 slices tomato and 4 tablespoons hummus
SNACK: Grilled Mixed Vegetables*
DINNER: Chicken Cranberry Nut Salad*
DESSERT: Chef Ronnda's Sexy Strawberry Walnut Dessert*
WATER: Half your body weight in ounces

TODAY'S WORKOUT

BACK, BI'S, AND THIGHS (CIRCUIT B); CORE; STRETCH-IT-OUT
Refer to Part 5 for specific exercises and correct form.

This is your fourth time doing Circuit B. Are you confident in your form and technique? Can you take it to the next level? Make sure you are maintaining good form during the stretches and that you concentrate on long breaths in and out while you are holding the stretch. And don't forget to do your stretches in the warm-up and cooldown.

REFUELING YOUR MUSCLE CELLS WITH FAT

During a circuit training workout that is medium to high in intensity your muscles are using a combination of sugar and fat as a fuel source, but predominantly sugar, because of the intensity level. Of course we all want to burn fat, so in order to maximize the amount of fat used to refuel

LOOK GOOD AND FEEL GOOD

Like many people, Alan Watson lives a busy life—he is a husband, father, and airline pilot. His goal was to get his body into the best shape possible so he would look good and feel good.

"I work hard and I enjoy life, and sometimes that involves a few beers and a great meal," admits Alan. "Working out four to five times a week and moderating my alcohol and portion sizes have been the keys to success for me. I was able to take off 22 pounds and 8 inches, with most of it coming from my waist. I have more energy, look good, am in good health, and feel great!"

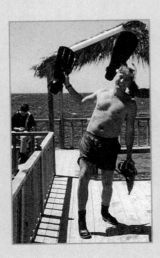 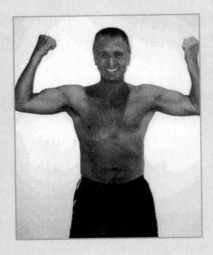

muscle cells, your blood sugar level and body chemistry have to be just right. You will refuel 50 to 60 percent of the calories you burned during your workout within the first two hours afterward. This means that if you burned 600 calories of sugar from your muscle cells in your circuit training workout, then 300 to 360 calories will be refueled into your muscle cells within the first two hours after your workout is over. Your goal is to burn off as much fat as possible, so when the workout is over it is important to hydrate your body with water during the first two hours and not consume any simple carbohydrates like juices or fruits that your body would use to refuel. In order to slow down the absorption of sugar into the bloodstream, you will want to eat a balanced meal of protein, healthy fats, and high-fiber carbohydrates. Remember, your goal is to burn fat, so you want to create the best possible environment in your body for that to happen.

Daily Reflection

On this day, answer the following questions in your journal:

1. Is there something in my life that I am wasting energy dwelling on? Is there something positive I can learn from this situation?
2. What do I tend to complain about the most? How can I change my approach so that I don't complain and waste precious energy?
3. What am I proud of myself for doing today?
4. What do I love about myself today?
5. What was the most rewarding part of my day?

DAY 14

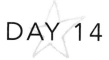

The three hardest tasks in the world are neither physical feats nor intellectual achievements, but moral acts: to return love for hate, to include the excluded, and to say, "I was wrong."
—*Sydney J. Harris, American journalist*

Today you are going to try your best to turn a negative situation into a positive one. When negative energy has an opportunity to build up in your mind, body, and soul, you are giving it the chance to be destructive to your health. Use your power to turn hate into love and cruelty into kindness whenever possible, and see it as a way to protect your health. Just think about how you feel after an argument compared to how you feel after giving someone a big hug and wishing them well. The argument drains energy from your body and leaves you feeling depressed and sad, whereas the giving gesture of a hug leaves you in positive good spirits. The next time you get into an argument, stop and ask yourself: is it better to be right, or better to be healthy in mind, body, and soul? Releasing love and kindness into the universe is guaranteed to make you a happier person.

> *Today's Affirmation*
> I will return love for hate, I will include the excluded, and I
> will have the courage to admit when I am wrong.

TODAY'S FOOD

Indulge! On this day of rest, you may want to enjoy a meal that is not on the meal plan. Once a week it is important to have a meal, dessert, or snack that you want just for the taste. Remember, moderation and portion control are still important!

The Menu

Recipes marked with an asterisk (*) can be found in the recipe section, Chapter 17.

BREAKFAST: Fast-and-Easy Poached Eggs*/Mixed Greens Salad* with 2 tablespoons cottage cheese/1 slice whole wheat toast with 1 tablespoon all-fruit blueberry jam

SNACK: ½ cup low-fat cottage cheese with ½ cup fresh berries

LUNCH: Curried Chicken Sandwich*

SNACK: ½ of a Turkey Pita Sandwich*

SNACK: 1 pear/1 piece of string organic low-fat cheese

DINNER: Fish Tacos*/Garlic Spinach*

DESSERT: 1 cup sliced strawberries and diced mango with a dollop of Greek yogurt

WATER: Half your body weight in ounces

TODAY'S WORKOUT

Rest, Relax, and Rejuvenate

Have you ever noticed that when you are experiencing anxiety, stress, or anger, you usually have a shallow quick breath, whereas when you are sitting by the ocean watching the sunset or resting on a massage table your breath is deep and slow? Taking deep breaths can help your body slow down and relax.

Eastern philosophies of health and well-being emphasize the balance of an invisible vital energy in the body, known as *qi*, pronounced *chee*. When a person is healthy, *qi* flows smoothly along channels in the body known as meridians. The flow of *qi* depends on the balance of two complementary yet opposing forces: *yin* and *yang*. When *yin* and *yang* are imbalanced in the body from stress, inactivity, anxiety, poor eating habits, or spiritual neglect, energy flow through the meridians becomes blocked and causes symptoms of illness.

Go through the following steps to experience the calming effects of deep breathing:

1. Find a comfortable place to sit: chair, floor, yoga mat, pillow, or bed.
2. Close your eyes, place your hands on your stomach, and take in a nice deep breath; feel your diaphragm expand as your lungs fill with air. Exhale and empty all the air out of your lungs. Feel a sense of relief in your mind and your body with each exhale.
3. Keep the air movement slow and continuous.
4. Try not to hold your breath; instead, gradually build up the length of each exhalation until you have reached 6 or 7 seconds.
5. Think of each exhalation as a release of the negative energy, stress, and anxiety out of your body and into the universe, leaving you the opportunity to rebalance the energy within your body.

Daily Reflection

On this day, answer the following questions in your journal:

1. What are three things that I can do to relax and how can I begin to implement them into my life?
2. What are some signs of imbalance in my daily life? For example, not eating properly, consuming too much caffeine, feeling stress and anxiety, working too much, not getting

enough relaxation, and/or not spending enough time with family. What steps can I take to rebalance my vital energy (*qi*)?

3. What three methods can I use to release negative energy from my body?
4. What do I love about myself?
5. What am I proud of myself for doing today?
6. Did I truly take a day off to rest? Is it possible to arrange my schedule for a day of rest?

DAY 15

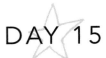

We may encounter many defeats but we must not be defeated.

—*Maya Angelou*

You must keep a winning spirit and learn from the valleys of life you may find yourself in when a relationship ends or when you lose a job, fail a test, or miss out on an opportunity. Life is a roller-coaster ride of highs and lows; when you are experiencing a low it's an opportunity to take a look at how you may be able to improve yourself for your future experience. You have to stay strong and realize that there will be other high points in your life; otherwise you risk staying in the valleys for too long, which can be detrimental to your health. Feeling defeated is like inviting depression in. Stay strong, and learn constructively from your experiences. Every failure or defeat is an opportunity to learn something new for next time. Never let your spirit become defeated.

> *Today's Affirmation*
> I may encounter many defeats throughout my life, but I will never be defeated.

TODAY'S FOOD

SUGAR AND THE FAT-BURNING PROCESS

Your body's preferred source of fuel is glycogen, which is made primarily from sugar or carbohydrates. Your body will always burn sugar first, then fat, and, as a last resort, protein. Since

SUGAR CONTENT OF SOME POPULAR SNACK FOODS

Snickers Bar	30 grams
2 cups orange juice	40 grams
3 Double Stuf Oreo cookies	39 grams
1 can Pepsi or Coke	39 grams
8 ounces Jamba Juice Smoothie Berry Bliss	31.3 grams

SUGAR CONTENT OF HOLLYWOOD TRAINER–SUGGESTED SNACK FOODS

1 orange	12 grams
1 cup Greek yogurt with ½ cup fresh berries and ¼ cup low-fat granola	15 grams
½ cup cottage cheese and ½ tomato	2 grams
1 apple and 1 string low-fat organic cheese	14 grams
Whole wheat crackers and cheese string	0 grams

your goal is to burn as much fat as possible, make sure you do your best to limit your sugar intake to less than 13 to 20 grams of sugar per meal or snack as well as throughout the day so you can keep your body burning fat all day.

The Menu

Recipes marked with an asterisk (*) can be found in the recipe section, Chapter 17.

BREAKFAST: Muscle Oats*

SNACK: ½ cup low-fat cottage cheese with 1 medium tomato, sliced, and seasoned with ground black pepper

LUNCH: Turkey Burger*

SNACK: Tomato Cucumber Salad*

SNACK: 1 orange

DINNER: Poached Wild Salmon*/Mixed Greens Salad*

DESSERT: Dark Chocolate–Covered Strawberries*
WATER: Half your body weight in ounces

TODAY'S WORKOUT

CARDIO BURN; STRETCH-IT-OUT
Refer to Part 5 for specific cardio exercises and form.

THE FAT-BURNING ZONE

Several pieces of cardio equipment claim they can tell you when you are working in your fat-burning zone, but the truth is, your fat-burning zone is specific to *you* and will depend on *your individual genetics and your fitness level,* things no exercise machine can take into account. This is why I recommend that you get an active metabolic test and use a heart rate monitor that you can program with all of your personal information. The manufacturers of these cardio machines choose a low-intensity range as a fat-burning zone to motivate the general population to improve their aerobic base. When you do cardio exercise at a low intensity, you will generally use more fat than sugar as a fuel source because your body has the ability to supply enough oxygen to your working muscles to break down fat. When you increase the intensity of your workout, your muscles' need for oxygen increases and, depending on your level of fitness, your body may not be able to take in enough oxygen to support the demand. This is when your body starts working anaerobically (without oxygen) and in turn burns more sugar as an energy source. Your body will never be in a 100 percent fat-burning state, because some will be reserved for your brain and nervous system, which require sugar/carbohydrates as a fuel source. You can find out how efficiently your body uses fat as a fuel source at specific heart rates by having an active metabolic test administered by a health-care professional. The more you know, the more you can tailor your program to work for you.

Take a moment to review the major points of your walking, jogging, running, or sprinting form introduced in Part 3: breathing, posture, stride length, push-off, recruiting your core muscles, pumping arms, and intention. And remember to fill in your Cardio Training Log.

LOWERING CHOLESTEROL THE DRUG-FREE WAY

Denise looked healthy from the outside, but like millions of people she had high cholesterol. She started the program with the simple goal of flattening the pouch on her lower belly, and after just six weeks lost 15 pounds and sculpted her body. She lost 5 percent body fat, and everyone has recognized the changes in her physique.

"I reached my goal of a flat stomach," boasts Denise, "but the best news is that when I went for a checkup, my doctor could not believe how much my cholesterol had gone down. In just six weeks it had dropped from 220 to 181."

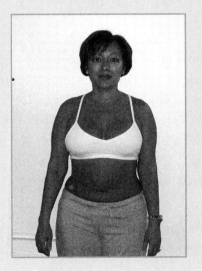 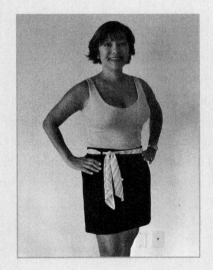

Daily Reflection

On this day, answer the following questions in your journal:

1. When is the last time I felt defeat or experienced a valley?
2. What two life lessons have I learned from my last valley?

3. What two things can I do to get through a valley?

4. What do I love about myself?

5. What did I learn from the second week that will help me improve my nutrition and workout program?

DAY 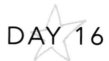 16

I was brought up to believe that how I saw myself was more important than how others saw me.
—*Anwar el-Sadat*

Don't let other people's views and opinions limit your life. Many times people are afraid to try something new because they don't want to be judged. Think about all the experiences you missed out on because you were concerned about what other people would think of you. Were you afraid to wear a bathing suit, so you didn't get to feel the refreshing water? Perhaps you were afraid to go onto the dance floor, so you missed out on that salsa lesson. Not anymore. It is time to live for yourself and step outside the box! People who love you for who you are will enjoy your spirit and seeing you happy! It's time to do *you*!

> *Today's Affirmation*
> How I see myself is more important than how others see me!

EXPAND YOUR HORIZONS

Variety is the spice of life. Trying something new takes self-confidence and courage, and is a great way to break a rut if you start to feel bored or uninspired by your workouts. Be courageous and add a new activity to your life. Here are some things you can add to your routine:

1. Join a club: running, swimming, triathlon, skiing, hiking, surfing, rock climbing, tennis, squash, badminton, golf, soccer, football, basketball, marathon, rowing, boxing, or martial arts. There are all kinds of sporting clubs that are very social and welcome

people at all levels of fitness. This is a great place to meet new people or families who are interested in active living. Many of these clubs have specific beginner programs, so don't be scared to get involved.

2. Take a class at a private studio devoted to yoga, Pilates, martial arts, indoor cycling, or dancing.

3. Take a private lesson in something new to decrease your fears and see if you would like it.

TODAY'S FOOD

BUZZ WORDS

Light, fat-free, sugar-free, heart-healthy, all-natural, low-sodium, cholesterol-free—these are just some of the phrases that manufacturers use to make you believe their products are good for you. It's up to *you* to understand what these things mean so you don't get duped. The place you will find the most important information is the ingredients list. Remember, the items that appear at the top of the list are the ones in the highest quantities. Therefore, if sugar, sucrose, fructose, corn syrup, molasses, high-fructose corn syrup, or any other "-ose" word is within the top six or seven ingredients, beware and compare.

Compare the ingredients labels on organic items with those on conventional foods and you will see a dramatic difference. Chances are that you'll recognize most of the ingredients in organic products. They are real foods that occur naturally on earth. On the other hand, the nonorganic foods have ingredients that you probably can't even pronounce, let alone recognize. These are chemical additives and preservatives that your body doesn't need or want.

Here's a short glossary of some of the terms you have to be aware of when you're grocery shopping for a healthy lifestyle:

Light: Even with less fat per serving, a "light" food can still be very high in calories and can contain chemicals and preservatives.

Fat-free: The food contains no fat, but look for chemical fat substitutes and sugar content.

Sugar-free: A no-sugar food may contain man-made chemical sugar substitutes.

Heart-healthy: Low in cholesterol and saturated fat, a heart-healthy food can be refined or processed, which is still bad for your heart

All-natural: The product is not man-made, but it can still have added chemicals to preserve it.

Cholesterol-free: A cholesterol-free food can still contain high amounts of sugar, sodium, additives, and preservatives.

Low-sodium: The food contains 140 mg or less of sodium per serving.

Certified Organic: This is the only label that guarantees there are no chemical additives or preservatives; it does not mean unprocessed. So it is still important to read the ingredients to find the best brands and products, those that are high in fiber. Remember, if it is wrapped, canned, or in a box it is probably processed.

The Menu

Recipes marked with an asterisk (*) can be found in the recipe section, Chapter 17.

BREAKFAST: Nutty Banana Protein Smoothie*
SNACK: 2 hard-boiled eggs, mashed and seasoned with a dash of salt and ground black pepper
LUNCH: Grilled Chicken Breasts*/1 cup steamed vegetables/½ cup brown rice
SNACK: Lemon Green Beans*
SNACK: Black Bean and Corn Salad*
DINNER: Chicken Fajitas* /1 cup steamed broccoli
DESSERT: 1 cup sliced peaches (fresh or canned in natural juice) with ½ cup low-fat vanilla yogurt
WATER: Half your body weight in ounces

DETOX AND FINE-TUNE

Heather came to me because she had tried a couple of different fitness programs but wasn't getting the results she was looking for. Like many people, she was focused on her weight to the point that it caused stress, which made it more difficult for her body to burn fat. Stress and weight loss are not compatible partners.

"Jeanette brought to my attention that I needed to cleanse my body to get rid of the toxins so I could try to bring back my hormonal balance," recalls Heather. "Like so many others, I treated stress and depression with prescription drugs, and each one had its own set of side effects. I spoke with my doctors and we all agreed that it would be okay for me to decrease my prescriptions to help detox my body. I also started to spend time volunteering. It helped my spirit to give love to other people who needed it and made me realize how blessed and fortunate I was. Of course, I work out five to six times a week and that is my natural drug, my daily happy-hormone high. I eat five to six small meals a day composed of fresh organic whole foods, and I feel great. I have gone down three dress sizes, and my friends and family are watching my body reshape before their eyes!"

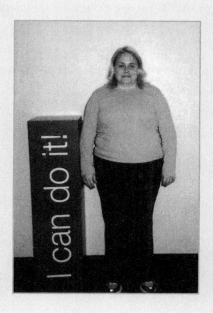
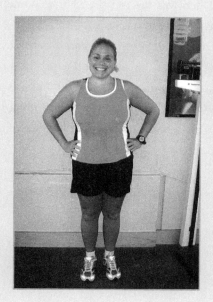

TODAY'S WORKOUT

CHEST, TRI'S, AND BOOTY (CIRCUIT A); CORE; STRETCH-IT-OUT
Refer to Part 5 for specific exercises and correct form.

TIGHT BOOTY!

One of the questions that I hear most often from both men and women is, "What are the best exercises to firm up my booty?" The top booty-shaping exercises are the single leg squat, the reverse lunge, back kicks, squats, and the single leg reach.

Daily Reflection

On this day, answer the following questions in your journal:

1. When was the last time I tried something new? What are three new things that I would like to try?
2. On what date and time can I try three new things?
3. When was the last time I was afraid to try something for fear other people would watch or judge me? How can I defeat the fear and build my confidence?
4. What am I proud of myself for doing today?
5. What was the most rewarding part of the day?

DAY 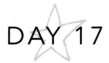 17

We gain strength, and courage, and confidence by each experience in which we really
stop to look fear in the face . . . we must do that which we think we cannot.
—*Eleanor Roosevelt*

Most people limit themselves before anyone else even has the opportunity to say no or turn them down. Fear will stop you from trying new things and enjoying life to the fullest. Always remember:

if you can conceive it, then you can achieve it. If you have the ability to imagine what you would like to do, then it's possible. All you have to do is get up off your butt and do it. Yes, you are going to hit roadblocks—rejection, jealousy, people who don't believe in you. But all of those experiences will make you stronger. By the time you reach your goals, you will have new ones that will come with their own set of fears, but this is how we grow. Welcome the discomfort that comes from fear as an opportunity to learn more about yourself. You will be surprised to see how strong and exciting you really are. How will you know if you don't give yourself a chance?

> *Today's Affirmation*
> I will not be afraid to try new things. I realize that I will only limit my own life experiences if I live in fear. I will gain strength, courage, confidence, and experience every time I step outside my comfort zone.

TODAY'S FOOD

HEALTHY MILK FROM HEALTHY COWS

You can only get healthy milk from a healthy cow! Many women who are going through menopause are told by their physicians to be cautious with or possibly limit their intake of dairy products because of the hormones used on cows. Choose organic milk that is taken from animals that have been grass fed and have had no hormones added. Even better, you may want to select real milk that is not pasteurized. Pasteurization is a process that kills off all the bacteria in milk, but the problem is, it also kills off the abundant *healthy* bacteria. Today there are better ways to ensure that our milk is free of disease-causing bacteria, one of which is for dairy farmers to treat their cows better and clean up their farming methods. If you are interested in helping to send conventional dairy farmers a message and saying no to pasteurized milk, you can find out where to get real organic unpasteurized milk that contains its own natural healthy bacteria at www.realmilk.com.

The Menu

· ·

Recipes marked with an asterisk (*) can be found in the recipe section, Chapter 17.

BREAKFAST: Guilt-Free Breakfast Quesadilla*

SNACK: 6 ounces Greek yogurt and ½ cup fresh berries garnished with 3 tablespoons of low-fat granola

LUNCH: Tuna Salad Wrap*

SNACK: 1 cup steamed broccoli

SNACK: 1 brown-rice cake with ½ cup low-fat cottage cheese and 2 tomato slices seasoned with a dash of ground black pepper

DINNER: Chinese Chicken Salad*

DESSERT: Apple Crisp*

WATER: Half your body weight in ounces

TODAY'S WORKOUT

CARDIO BURN; STRETCH-IT-OUT

Refer to Part 5 for specific exercises. And, today, be sure to hold those stretches for 1 to 3 minutes.

HIGH INTENSITY DOESN'T MEAN HIGH IMPACT

High intensity is a term used to describe a workout that is very challenging. A high-intensity workout will push you to your limits, and you will be working at a heart rate above 75 percent of your max for most of the session.

High impact describes the amount of stress a workout will put on your joints. High-impact activities are those that have you jumping or taking both feet off of the ground at the same time, things like running, jumping jacks, jump squats, jump lunges, tennis, basketball, running stairs, sprinting, some dance moves (including certain aerobic dance moves), and some kickboxing moves. It is not safe for overweight people to participate in high-impact activities, but this doesn't mean they can't get a great workout. There are many types of exercise that are high intensity but low impact, such as swimming and cycling. So don't confuse intensity with impact.

If you are very overweight it is best to decrease your body weight and strengthen your joints with low-impact activities and strength training before moving into the high-impact exercises.

Always exercise smart. You don't have to jump up and down to get an effective workout. You have the power to control the impact and intensity of your workouts so that you are getting the best results for you.

MINDFUL EATING

I met Noemy while taping *Weighing In* for the Food Network. An avid runner, she was training for her fifth marathon. She was disciplined with her training regimen but unhappy with her weight. Noemy is not alone; many of my clients come to me advanced in terms of fitness but still unhealthy in terms of diet. Without the second half of the equation, i.e., a balanced and nutritious diet, you're never going to be completely healthy. "The most important thing I learned from Jeanette was that proper eating is a science," says Noemy. "You can cheat yourself on the diet, but you can't cheat the laws of science. The hardest unhealthy habit to break was eating without thinking. When I stop and think, I remember the lifestyle I want to live—to be healthy and thin. Conscious eating helps me avoid what my body doesn't need. I have found healthy alternatives, but it is still a daily challenge to be mindful when I eat."

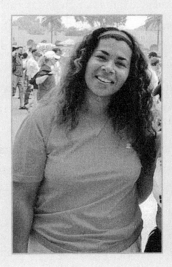 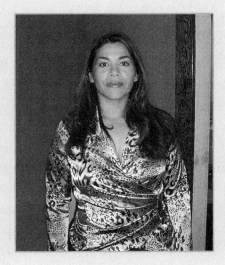

Daily Reflection

On this day, answer the following questions in your journal:

1. What are two things that I have always wanted to do but was too afraid to try?
2. What will I gain and what will I lose if I try one of these activities?
3. What will I gain from feeling uncomfortable and fearful?
4. What am I proud of myself for doing today?

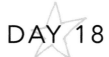

DAY 18

More than anything else, I believe it's our decisions,
not the conditions of our lives, that determine our destiny.
—*Anthony Robbins*

People love to use excuses when it comes to explaining why they are overweight and out of shape: a slow metabolism, a messed-up thyroid, a genetic predisposition, can't afford a gym membership, don't have day care, have to work, bad knee, asthma . . . the list is endless. There is no excuse. No matter what your circumstances, there are ways to live a healthy life. Remember who you are dealing with here. I was raised in government housing on powdered milk, around lots of impoverished, single moms and battered children—I've seen and heard it all. Yes, there are some stories that are more painful than others, but why make it a competition? It's time to take responsibility for your life, and use your experiences to make you smarter and stronger.

My clients who have accepted that they are responsible for their health have a much higher success rate. They recognize that if they had the power to become overweight and out of shape, they also have the power to turn their lives around. Those who have not taken responsibility spend a lot of time making excuses and don't believe in their own power to change. They are so busy looking everywhere else for the answer that they fail to look in the mirror.

It's time to face the truth: no one hid the ingredients list on a box of cookies from you. You chose not to read them. No one barred you from the grocery store. You chose to eat out. No one forced that soda down your throat. You chose to drink it. And no one cut your legs off. You decided not to use them!

The purpose of getting you to accept responsibility for your state of health is to get you to understand that power you used to degrade your health is the same power you can use to improve your health.

> *Today's Affirmation*
> The decisions that I make will determine my future and my destiny!

TODAY'S FOOD

ACTIVE BACTERIA CULTURES

Make sure to look for active bacteria cultures when you choose your yogurt. Some of the most common active bacteria cultures that you may find in yogurt are: L. bulgaricus, S. thermophilus, L. acidophilus, Bifidum, L. casei, and L. reuteri. Active or beneficial bacteria are also known as probiotics, and although they occur naturally in our digestive tracts they need regular replenishing. Studies show that active bacteria improve intestinal function, promote good digestive health, and enhance our body's defenses against a number of ailments.

The Menu

Recipes marked with an asterisk (*) can be found in the recipe section, Chapter 17.

BREAKFAST: Greek Yogurt Crunch*
SNACK: 2 hard-boiled eggs, mashed and seasoned with a dash of salt and ground black pepper
LUNCH: Turkey BLT Pita Pocket*
SNACK: Broccoli Parmesan*
SNACK: 1 brown-rice cake with 1 tablespoon soy nut butter and ½ tablespoon all-fruit blueberry jam

AFTER GASTRIC BYPASS

Tanya was introduced to me by the producers of *The Tyra Banks Show* when they requested my help to condition Tanya's heart in order to prepare her for additional surgery needed to remove the excess skin hanging off her body following a gastric bypass.

"When I started working with Jeanette I could only last five minutes on the treadmill walking at a speed of 2.5 miles per hour," admits Tanya. "As I began to work out on a regular basis and eat healthy I started to feel much better about myself and my future. I have suffered many side effects from gastric bypass surgery, including acid reflux, pain in my abdomen and stomach, scars, and bouts of depression. Surgery did not improve the condition of my heart, lungs, and muscles, and if I could do it all over again I would choose to change my lifestyle instead of having surgery. I now feel like I have a new lease on life. If you can still walk I highly recommend that you choose exercise and healthy eating instead of surgery. I can now do intervals of running and walking for three miles nonstop and I feel great!"

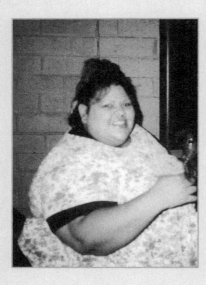
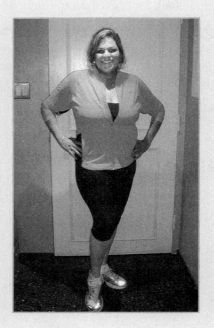

DINNER: Broiled Lemon-Garlic Sea Bass*/Cranberry Walnut Salad*
DESSERT: 1 cup sliced strawberries and bananas
WATER: Half your body weight in ounces

TODAY'S WORKOUT

BACK, BI'S, AND THIGHS (CIRCUIT B); CORE; STRETCH-IT-OUT
Refer to Part 5 for specific exercises and correct form.

LOW INTENSITY DOESN'T MEAN LOW IMPACT

A low-intensity workout is one that is going to be easy to moderately challenging, meaning your heart rate will stay below 75 percent of your max for the entire workout.

A low-impact workout is one that is going to put less stress on your joints although it can still be high in intensity. Low impact does not mean easy, it just means less stress on your joints by always keeping one foot in contact with the ground. Some great forms of low-impact exercise for beginners are power walking, swimming, aquafitness, elliptical machine, walking stairs/Stairmaster, cycling, cross-country skiing, Nordic track, low-impact aerobics classes, body sculpting, weight training, Pilates, gentle yoga, boxing or kickboxing without jumping, and dancing without jumping. You have the power to control the intensity and impact of workouts for your maximum benefit.

Daily Reflection

On this day, answer the following questions in your journal:

1. What are two decisions that I am going to make today to change my destiny?
2. How am I going to implement these new decisions into my life?
3. What decisions have I made in the past that I am most proud of?
4. What was the most rewarding part of the day?

DAY 19

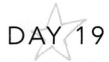

The function of education is to teach one to think intensively and to think critically . . .
intelligence plus character—that is the goal of true education.

—*Martin Luther King, Jr.*

The multimillion-dollar health, fitness, and nutrition industries are, first and foremost, in the business of making profits. If you benefit from their products and services, that's good. But it is your responsibility to educate yourself on anything that has to do with your body, whether it's a pharmaceutical, a supplement, or food item. You need to understand how they are going to affect your life and what side effects you may have in the short term and the long term. Remember, the salesperson is only going to divulge all of the great things about it. So use all the resources available to find out the details that they may not be telling you. You should question everything, no matter what the source. Build a network of health professionals whom you trust. It is better to ask questions than to be ignorant. (A list of resources to help you appears in the back of this book. You can also consult my Web site www.thehollywoodtrainer.com.)

> *Today's Affirmation*
> I will continue to think intensively and critically. I will continue to educate myself through reading, asking questions, and analyzing my life experiences. The more educated I am about health, fitness, and nutrition, the better prepared I will be to make healthy lifestyle decisions for myself and my family.

TODAY'S FOOD

KNOW YOUR GRAINS

Sprouted wheat is the healthiest way to get whole grains. The whole wheat kernel is literally sprouted. As a wheat kernel grows, many vitamins are formed, which means that products made with sprouted wheat have added nutritional value. You can buy delicious breads made with sprouted wheat at your local health food store or in many supermarkets.

Whole grain means that both parts of the grain, the bran and the germ, are included. The bran and the germ are the most nutrient-rich parts of the grain; thus whole-grain products are far healthier than products made with refined white flour. Whole grain can refer to any kind of grain, including spelt and kamut.

Whole wheat is used when you are referring specifically to common wheat grain, and again, is healthier than anything made with white flour.

Gluten is a protein that is found in wheat. All products that contain wheat also contain gluten. Some people experience heavy stomach bloating after eating wheat products. If this is the case, you may want to try eating gluten-free products and getting tested for allergies.

Spelt is an ancient grain genetically related to wheat but is a completely different species than modern-day wheat. Spelt has a unique "nutty" flavor and is a highly nutritious alternative to traditional wheat grain. If you are allergic to gluten, you may be able to eat bread products made from spelt.

The Menu

Recipes marked with an asterisk (*) can be found in the recipe section, Chapter 17.

BREAKFAST: Blueberry and Banana Buckwheat Pancakes*/Chef Ronnda's Turkey Sausage Patties*
SNACK: 1 apple
LUNCH: Mom's Turkey Vegetable Chili *
SNACK: Baked Butternut Squash*
SNACK: One 6-inch whole wheat pita pocket bread stuffed with 4 slices tomatoes and 4 tablespoons hummus
DINNER: Greek Chicken Salad*
DESSERT: 2 Oatmeal Raisin Cookies*
WATER: Half your body weight in ounces

GET YOUR BODY BACK—MOMMY-AND-ME STYLE!

Kimberly had a beautiful baby girl, but during her pregnancy she gained more than 60 pounds. Because she works as a professional model and actress, it was imperative that Kimberly get back in shape so she could work again.

"As soon as I got the okay from my doctor, I started walking every day with my baby girl," Kimberly recalls. "After a few weeks I began to regain my strength and stamina, and added resistance training and Pilates to my weekly workout program. Like every new mom, I did not want to leave my baby for even five minutes. So I did my best to incorporate my daughter into my workouts and that way I could still spend time with her. After six months of eating healthy, walking with the stroller, doing Pilates, and playing Mommy-and-me games, I was able to get my body back."

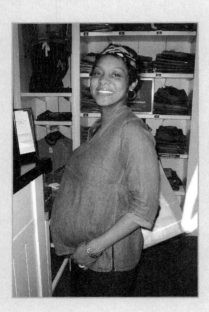 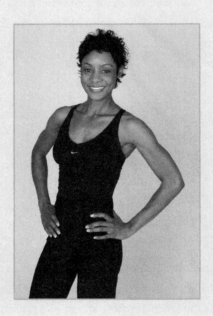

TODAY'S WORKOUT

CHEST, TRI'S, AND BOOTY (CIRCUIT A); STRETCH-IT-OUT
Refer to Part 5 for specific exercises and correct form.

Now that you've been at it for a couple of weeks, how long does it take you to do Circuit A from beginning to end? Time yourself and make a note in your journal, comparing it to your times from the first two weeks. Remember, your form has to be good and you can't rush through the exercises. Remember too that each set has a number of repetitions between 10 and 25. A set may also be an isometric hold for 30 seconds like the plank or squat/chair pose.

UNDERARM FLAB

Want to get rid of that underarm flab? Excellent exercises to help firm up the backs of your arms are push-ups, planks, dips, overhead triceps extensions, overhead shoulder presses, triceps kick-backs, triceps press downs on a cable machine, and boxing.

Daily Reflection

On this day, answer the following questions in your journal:

1. Who are two references (a person, Web site, chat room, or health-care facility) that I can use when I have a question related to nutrition?
2. Who are two references that I can use when I have a question related to exercise?
3. Who can I call when I have questions related to my health?
4. What have I done today that I am proud of?
5. What was the most rewarding part of the day?

DAY 20

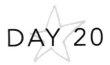

Men often become what they believe themselves to be. If I believe I cannot do something,
it makes me incapable of doing it. But when I believe I can, then I acquire
the ability to do it even if I didn't have it in the beginning.
—Mahatma Gandhi

It's time to remember your self-fulfilling prophecy. You can do it! Believing in yourself is one of the most important factors in achieving success. Throughout your journey to improve your health and change your body you will experience challenges that you will be able to overcome only through believing. You have to believe in your strength and ability to succeed. As long as you believe in yourself you will reach your goal.

> *Today's Affirmation*
> I believe that I can exercise and eat healthy every day to improve the quality of my life.

TODAY'S FOOD

LYCOPENE

Lycopene is an antioxidant found in tomatoes, guava, rose hip, watermelon, and pink grapefruit. Research shows that lycopene in tomatoes can be absorbed more efficiently by the body if processed into juice, sauce, or paste. High intake of lycopene-containing fruits and vegetables will decrease your risk of certain types of cancer. Habitual intake of tomato products has been associated with a decreased risk of cancer of the digestive tract among Italians. In one six-year study by Harvard Medical School and Harvard School of Public Health, the diets of more than 47,000 men were studied; of forty-six fruits and vegetables evaluated, only the tomato products showed a measurable relationship to a reduced risk of prostate cancer. As consumption of tomato products increased, levels of lycopene in the blood increased, and the risk of prostate cancer decreased. The study also showed that the heat needed to process tomatoes and tomato products increases lycopene's bioavailability. Ongoing research suggests that lycopene is also associated with reduced risk of macular degenerative disease, serum lipid oxidation, and cancers of the lung, bladder, cervix, and skin.

The Menu

* *

Recipes marked with an asterisk (*) can be found in the recipe section, Chapter 17.

BREAKFAST: Egg BLT Pita Pocket*
SNACK: 1 pear and 1 string organic low-fat cheese
LUNCH: 1½ cups low-sodium tomato soup/Mixed Greens Salad*
SNACK: Asian Chicken–Cabbage Salad*
SNACK: ½ cup low-fat cottage cheese with ½ cup fresh berries
DINNER: Honey-Mustard Lamb Chops*/Roasted Asparagus*/Honey-Glazed Carrots*
DESSERT: Chef Ronnda's Almond Ricotta Cheesecake*
WATER: Half your body weight in ounces

TODAY'S WORKOUT

BACK, BI'S, AND THIGHS (CIRCUIT B); CORE; STRETCH-IT-OUT
Refer to Part 5 for specific exercises and correct form, and incorporate the stretches during the warm-up and cooldown.

HIGH-INTENSITY AND LOW-INTENSITY WORKOUTS

It's important to vary a fitness routine with both high- and low-intensity exercises because both have benefits for fat burning, weight loss, and overall health. Low-intensity workouts that gradually increase in intensity over time will help you build your aerobic base. When you build your aerobic base you become more efficient at using fat as a fuel source and you will be able to participate in high-intensity workouts without feeling nauseated or light-headed. High-intensity workouts help you increase the amount of calories that you burn and will increase your metabolic rate, especially for the first two hours after your workout is complete. High-intensity workouts put a greater demand on your muscles, which will create a greater physical response. Both styles of workouts are important and both will help you burn fat, burn calories, and change your physique!

BREAKING A PLATEAU

I met Barbara at a Delta Sigma Theta Sorority Health Summit in Jamaica cosponsored by the BET Foundation. Barbara, who had already started her journey to a new healthy life, was participating in Delta's weight-loss challenge and eager to get as much information as she could from speakers at the summit.

Back home, Barbara hired me to work with her, mostly because she'd hit a plateau in her training and was becoming discouraged. Together, we were able to break her plateau while learning and having a lot of fun along the way.

"In a short eight weeks working with Jeanette, I was able to lose an additional 22 pounds and two dress sizes," Barbara remembers. "Jeanette taught me that exercising at the right intensity levels along with proper nutrition would move me to the next level. People cannot stop talking about how my body is transforming right before their eyes. From the time I started my journey I have lost a total of 60 pounds and five dress sizes. I am feeling great and I know I will hit my goal of 144 pounds."

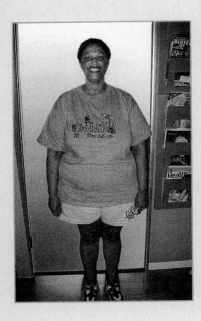 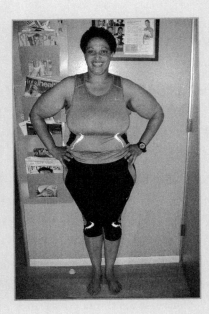

Daily Reflection

On this day, answer the following questions in your journal:

1. What do I love about myself today?
2. What am I proud of myself for doing today?
3. What was the most challenging part of today's program?
4. What can I do to overcome this challenge?

DAY 21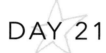

The very purpose of religion is to control yourself, not to criticize others. Rather, we must criticize
ourselves. How much am I doing about my anger? About my attachment, about my hatred,
about my pride, my jealousy? These are the things that we must check in daily life.
—*His Holiness the Dalai Lama*

When something causes you anxiety, anger, or stress, take a moment to write down your thoughts before you react. Think about what has triggered your negative feelings, and why a particular experience has led you to react the way you have. The process of writing down the experience and your feelings can help you release the stress, anger, or anxiety from your body so you can be at peace.

> ·   ·   · *Today's Affirmation* ·   ·   ·
> I will check myself daily to see what I am doing to control my anger,
> attachment, hatred, pride, and jealousy. My mind and spirit
> must be healthy if I want to strengthen my body and enjoy life.

TODAY'S FOOD

SHARING RECIPES

Take time to enjoy your food. Exchange recipes with friends, be creative with spices and flavors, and try dishes from various cultures. Food brings us great joy in life, and making healthy choices doesn't mean your meals shouldn't be flavorful and delicious.

The Menu

Recipes marked with an asterisk (*) can be found in the recipe section, Chapter 17.

BREAKFAST: Egg White–Turkey Scramble*

SNACK: 6 ounces Greek yogurt with ½ cup fresh berries, garnished with 3 tablespoons low-fat granola

LUNCH: Turkey Meatballs*/1 cup cooked whole wheat pasta with ¾ cup marinara sauce/ Mixed Greens Salad*

SNACK: 1 small pink grapefruit

SNACK: Pear–Pine Nut Salad*

DINNER: Apple Pork Tenderloin*/Garlic Rapini Potatoes*

DESSERT: California Fruit Salad*

WATER: Half your body weight in ounces

TODAY'S WORKOUT

REST, RELAX, AND REJUVENATE

When you are able to control your mind instead of allowing it to control you, then you will bring peace and harmony into your life.

MEDITATION THROUGH VISUALIZATION

Listening to music that replicates the sounds of nature, like chirping birds or crashing ocean waves, can help you visualize a relaxing place by engaging your sense of hearing. Here are simple steps to discover a whole new world right in your own home:

1. Find a comfortable place to sit and relax, like a chair, cushion, floor, or mat. Close your eyes and calm your body by breathing slowly and steadily.
2. Inhale and feel your lungs expand, then exhale and feel your body relax.
3. Close your eyes and hear the ocean rolling in and crashing against the shore.
4. Visualize the clear blue ocean, the colorful birds, and the tropical foliage.
5. Smell the scent of the healing salts from the ocean.
6. Feel the healing, invigorating sea air blowing across your skin, and the warmth of the sun penetrating your arms, legs, and face.
7. Enjoy this time, relax, be joyous, and continue to breathe.

PAMPER YOURSELF

1. Get a good night's sleep—naturally.
2. Have someone give you a massage.
3. Write down feelings to release them from your body.
4. Indulge in aromatherapy or a simple bubble bath.
5. Light incense and play relaxing music.
6. Take a walk close to nature.
7. Meditate.
8. Try a yoga, tai chi, or qi gong class (or follow a DVD).
9. Pray.
10. Attend or join a spiritual function at a church, temple, mosque, or other spiritual/religious institution.
11. Explore your inner artist: paint, take photographs, make jewelry, knit . . .
12. Enjoy a steam room, sauna, or Jacuzzi.
13. Take a day at a spa—even a "home spa."
14. Try acupuncture or reflexology.
15. Do your stretching exercises.
16. Spend a few moments being aware of your breathing.

Daily Reflection

On this day, answer the following questions in your journal:

1. What are two things that I can do to become a better person?
2. What are ten things that I love about myself?
3. What are three things that I can do to release negative energy from my body?
4. What was the most rewarding part of the past twenty-one days?
5. What was the most challenging part of the past twenty-one days?
6. What can I do to overcome this challenge?
7. How do I feel about my efforts over the past twenty-one days?

Congratulations! You have completed your first twenty-one days on the Hollywood Trainer Weight-Loss Plan. But don't stop here. . . . This is just the beginning of your new life. The next and final part of the book will give you a summary of the seven steps and the elements you need to make your own program so you can make healthy living a habit.

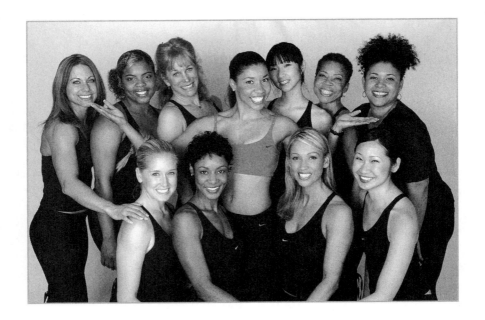

Part Four

EATING FOR LIFE

"Let food be your medicine and medicine be your food."

—*Hippocrates*

Here's your crash course in healthy eating, providing the fundamentals of what you need to know to get healthy once and for all. I cover topics from emotional eating to portion control, organic foods to diet sodas, with lots of practical guidance about what you can do today—and over time—to put what you're learning into action.

9

THE MENTAL AND EMOTIONAL
SIDE OF EATING

"Thou shouldst eat to live, not live to eat."

—*Socrates*

n keeping with the core principles of my plan, when it comes to nutrition I believe knowledge is power. You need to know how to make the right food choices so you don't feel frustrated when it is time to eat. Is this the right food? Is this the right time to eat it? Should I have fewer carbs and more protein? What about those healthy fats? Will they really help me lose weight? Should I eat a chicken burger without the bread? Are artificial sweeteners better then sugar?

You've probably tried one or more of the popular diets out there, lost some weight at first, then gained all of it—and sometimes more—back. What an emotional roller coaster! You're not alone in your frustrations. Millions of people experience various types of anxiety when it comes to mealtime. I recognize this is an important issue to address so you can handle any mental or emotional baggage related to your eating habits. It is time to educate yourself about the food that you put into your body. I hope that by the time you are done reading this section you will have the knowledge to put together healthy, delicious meals that taste good, help you burn fat, and leave you feeling strong—physically, mentally, and spiritually.

You can breathe easy, because the yo-yoing and frustration are all behind you. The holistic approach to healthy eating that I offer will continue to work for you long after you put this book down and long after you've completed the initial twenty-one-day plan. I recognize that you know how important it is to eat right, but I also know that life gets crazy and sometimes it just seems easier to order in your favorite take-out or stop by the fast-food drive-thru. The problem is, once you go back onto autopilot—not thinking or caring about the food you eat and ignoring the negative side effects to your health—it's too easy to keep doing it. Before you know it, you can't remember the last time you had something fresh and wholesome to eat and you're back to feeling sluggish, enervated, depressed, anxious, and overwhelmed. Oh yes! There is a direct relationship between what you eat and how you feel and look. Instead of using pharmaceuticals to lift you out of depression, try giving your brain, nervous system, and hormonal system the nutrients they need to function at their best. Healthy eating is not just for Olympic athletes trying to win gold, it is a necessity for you to function at your best! Aren't you sick and tired of feeling sick and tired?

Despite our best intentions, we still make bad choices when it comes to food. One of the primary reasons is emotional eating. When Socrates said, "Thou shouldst eat to live, not live to eat," more than 2,500 years ago, he probably did not anticipate the epidemic of "living to eat" in which we find ourselves today—and why two-thirds of us are overweight, and millions are suffering from diet-related diseases. Research from the Centers for Disease Control (2003–2004) reported that more than 132 million Americans over the age of twenty are either overweight or obese and that more than 12.5 million children and teens between the ages of two and nineteen are either overweight or obese. In fact, obesity is a global epidemic. In our world of relative comfort and plenty, we've completely lost touch with our bodies' *needs*, and have instead become all too attuned to their *wants*. Let's get one thing straight: we eat so that the highly complex machinery of our bodies can continue to function and support us as we go about our lives. But too often we turn to food for other reasons: to relieve loneliness or boredom or to alleviate stress or depression. And it's not uncommon for us to use the excuse of a happy occasion to celebrate with food and drink that's not good for us. Once you start using food as a crutch, you initiate a cycle of emotional eating that often leads to poor health, weight gain, and depression.

Emotional eating is a danger to all of us—we're all human, and sometimes ice cream really does make us feel better! But if you start to recognize a pattern in your behavior, like always overeating after a stressful day at work or bingeing whenever you have relationship problems, you need to address the underlying problems in a way that is not harmful to you. Often emotional eating disguises serious issues, and it's worth considering counseling or therapy if it will help you find peace somewhere other than in the fridge. Not only do you have the ability to stop the cycle, in fact, you're the *only* one who can.

You have the power to free yourself from the vicious cycle of emotional eating, and I am going to help you. First, I will educate you on the nutritional information you need to make the right food choices. Second, I will provide you with a meal plan and recipes so you have the step-by-step help to prepare your food every day and in the correct portion sizes. Third, you will complete the daily spiritual affirmations and journal questions in the twenty-one-day plan, so you can really *love yourself* and strengthen your mental and spiritual foundation. Finally, you will build a supportive environment of friends, therapists, support group, family, and faith so that when the going gets tough, the all-you-can-eat buffet does not turn into your best friend.

JEANETTE'S RX

If you are an "emotional eater," ask yourself these questions every time you eat:

1. *Why am I eating?*
   You should eat because you are hungry, not because you are sad, bored, or even happy, and certainly not because everyone around you is eating.
2. *What am I eating?*
   The food you eat should be wholesome and rich in nutrients, not junk or comfort food.
3. *How much am I eating?*
   Eat enough to satisfy you, not so much that you feel stuffed. Learn to listen to your body and know when you've had enough.

10

CHOOSING AND LOSING

L et's start with this simple truth: if you want to lose fat, start feeling great, and function at your absolute best, you *have* to choose to start eating healthier *now*. Your body requires nutrients—vitamins, minerals, essential fatty acids, protein, carbohydrates, water, light, and oxygen—in order to accomplish your goals.

These nutrients are rarely found in the fast and processed foods that we consume at an alarming rate. Think about how often you settle for a dinner option you know is unhealthy just because it's easier than cooking up something nutritious. I know, it happens; but if you continue to eat foods that are low in nutrients and high in processing chemicals, flavor enhancers, and preservatives, you're setting your body up to suffer. Millions of people are living with diabetes, high blood pressure, high cholesterol, and other ailments as a result of—or at least worsened by—making unhealthy food choices. Many of these people are also on medication for one or more of these ailments, with each prescription bringing its own set of side effects and risks. Pumping our bodies full of pills and chemicals as a corrective measure does not address the real source of our health issues—unhealthy food choices resulting in a poor diet. We don't have to be slaves to a health food store or a highly restricted diet. The solution to our health crisis is at our fingertips.

PORTION CONTROL:
WHEN LESS REALLY IS MORE

Aside from making unhealthy food choices, the other main reason we have an obesity crisis is our belief that bigger is better. We just eat too much. Order an entrée in almost any restaurant and nine times out of ten, it's big enough for at least two or three adults. (And no matter how big the portion, we have been conditioned from childhood to eat everything on our plates because children were starving in other parts of the world.) Most of us have no idea what constitutes an appropriate individual serving size, and so have no concept that by eating what's put in front of us, we're actually eating way past the point of necessity. When we eat too much, the stomach, which is made up of smooth muscle, gets stretched, and the appetite increases. So the more we eat too much, the more we will *continue* to eat too much. Restaurants and food marketers may have skewed our sense of normal portion size, but we have to recognize that lack of portion control and emotional eating can become a cycle that will lead down the path to poor health. So the next time you're served a giant entrée at your favorite restaurant, think of it as your next two meals—eat half and ask for the rest to be wrapped to take home. You'll get twice the satisfaction.

JEANETTE'S RX

With just a little planning, you can modify your eating schedule to accommodate six or seven small balanced meals a day instead of two or three big ones. Eating smaller meals more frequently will not expand the stomach muscles, and it allows for more stable blood sugar levels, reducing the risk of diabetes. You will also experience fewer cravings and appetite swings. Plus, it's good for your metabolism, as your body's furnace burns fat all day long, rather than letting the sluggish effects of low blood sugar take over.

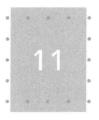

11

"WHOLE" FOODS

There's a lot of discussion about the meanings of *whole, natural, organic, unprocessed,* and a host of other terms that food marketers use nowadays. Throughout this section, I'll be referring to these terms as they are used to describe different kinds of "health" food and discussing what they mean to your food choices.

WHOLE FOODS

Food that is not processed or refined—or is minimally processed or refined—is generally referred to as *whole*. The term is a broad classification that includes both organic and conventional foods. Whole foods are high in vitamins, antioxidants, phytonutrients, minerals, and dietary fiber and include a wide variety of foods such as fresh fruits, vegetables, grains, cereals, beans, and legumes. They usually have a very short shelf life. The term *whole food* does not mean it is organic. Most grocery stores today carry conventional whole foods that have been genetically modified and treated with various chemicals to extend shelf life and fight off insects.

ORGANIC VERSUS CONVENTIONAL

Organic is a label applied to food that has been grown, harvested, and transported without the use of conventional pesticides, fertilizers, sewage sludge, bioengineering, or ionizing radiation. Organic meat, poultry, eggs, and dairy products come from animals that are given no antibiotics or growth hormones. Some organic farmers and manufacturers emphasize the use of renewable resources and environmental conservation. Before a product can be stamped with the official organic label, the farms and facilities the food comes from must pass inspection and receive certification. If a food bears the USDA organic stamp it is at least 95 percent organic. However, not all organic products are marked with this seal, so you must read package labels for chemicals and look out for signs or ask the staff at your local supermarket. Be aware of the term *natural,* which is not the same as *organic,* and that claims such as "free-range" and "hormone-free" can appear on products that are not organic.

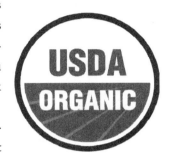

Although the USDA makes no claims that organic food is safer or more nutritious than conventional food, it's my firm belief that eating organic is better for you as well as for the environment. I personally follow a diet that is 80 to 90 percent organic, and not only do I feel great, but I also appreciate the superior quality and flavor of organic foods. Food and agriculture are big business, and a lot of the things you're buying in the supermarket have been produced by corporations that care far more about their profits than your health. Many people wait until they are suffering from cancer, acid reflux, irritable bowel syndrome, diabetes, or some other disease before they pay attention to the quality of their food; eating organic is one more way of taking control now, and ensuring that you are giving your body top-quality fuel.

PROCESSED VERSUS UNPROCESSED FOODS

The term *processed food* is thrown around all the time, but what does it actually mean? Processed food is food that has been altered from its natural whole state, destroying most of the valuable nutrients such as fiber, vitamins, minerals, phytonutrients, and antioxidants. Manufacturers treat food with chemical additives to extend its shelf life and/or to make it taste, look, and smell good. Any food that you buy in a can, jar, packet, or bottle is usually a processed food, although processed food comes in other kinds of packaging too.

THE CONSEQUENCES OF EATING REFINED AND PROCESSED FOODS

In the 1920s, researcher and dentist Dr. Weston Price and his wife, Monica Price, R.N., started noticing a sharp rise in tooth decay and degenerative disease diagnoses among their patients. In search of an explanation, they started to look at diet as a possible contributing factor. In order to test their theory, they conducted a nine-year study of the dietary practices of so-called "primitive" peoples—native groups and populations that subsisted entirely on indigenous foods. Of the fourteen tribal diets they studied, although radically different from one another, each provided an almost complete immunity to a range of illnesses, including cancer, tooth decay, heart disease, and diabetes. While these diets were diverse—some based on seafood, some on animal or dairy products, some on raw foods— they shared some noticeable characteristics. Perhaps most significant, none of the diets contained any processed, refined, or devitalized foods such as white sugar, white flour, canned foods, pasteurized or skim milk, or refined/hydrogenated vegetable oils. All contained some form of animal product and unrefined natural salt. (The native peoples would dry, salt, or ferment their food to preserve it, all of which methods conserve, or even increase, a food's inherent nutritional value.)

By following their traditional nature-based diets, these fourteen groups thrived in good health. However, as the Prices also discovered, those populations that had adopted diets including processed foods and refined sugar quickly developed a variety of health problems, including misshapen teeth and bones.

WHAT'S ADDED?

To enhance flavor and/or texture, manufacturers will simply pump food full of extra unhealthy fats, refined sugar, or salt, none of which you want in your body, and to extend shelf life, they add chemicals that do not occur naturally in food and that do not belong in your body.

It's been estimated that we each consume around five kilograms (eleven pounds) of food additives, such as preservatives, coloring, bleach, flavoring, flavor enhancers, emulsifiers, and stabilizers, every year. Consuming unnatural substances not only results in extra work for our bodies to break these chemicals down, but frequently triggers asthma attacks, rashes, respiratory irregularities, headaches, cancer, hyperactivity in children, and, in some, an abnormal sensitivity to medications, particularly aspirin.

Many people will cite studies that supposedly prove that additives are safe, but most of the tests that have been conducted have looked at the effects of just one additive during a limited time frame. There have been no definitive studies to date on the combined effect of large amounts of multiple chemical food additives over extended periods of time.

WHAT'S TAKEN AWAY?

Foods have a natural life span beyond which they lose their nutritive qualities; in nature, this renders them no longer fit for consumption, and they will decay, becoming food for insects and bacteria. When foods are pumped full of chemical additives, they will have an increased shelf life and remain technically consumable long after their naturally intended sell-by date. But those additives do nothing to preserve the food's nutrients, and so by the time you take it home and eat it, it will have little to no nutritional content left at all.

WHAT'S LEFT?

A whole lot of nothing! Processed food is largely comprised of chemical compounds and empty calories, which have all the staying power of unprocessed food calories but none of the energizing or nutritional qualities. Often the food industry will add vitamins and minerals to the foods they have processed to depletion, so you will see labels claiming that a food is "fortified with" one vitamin or mineral or another. This sounds good but, the truth is, fortifying food after it has been devitalized cannot duplicate the healthy, healing benefits derived from eating phytonutrients and phytochemicals in their naturally occurring combinations.

HOW PROCESSED FOOD MAKES YOU FAT

Last, but certainly not least, on the list of reasons to cut processed foods out of your diet is the fact that they erode your body's metabolism. Processed food is so highly refined that it is recognized by the body as sugar; when you eat these foods, your blood sugar level soars, triggering a massive release of the stabilizing hormone insulin. The problem is, any sudden rush of insulin into your system triggers your body's fat-storing mode as you try to conserve energy while the insulin does its job of removing the extra sugar from your blood. If you are eating processed foods two or three times a day, you are not only likely to gain weight, but you also considerably increase your risk of diabetes and metabolic syndrome.

The good news is that you don't have to eat this junk! Choose wholesome foods like brown rice, oatmeal, nuts, beans, fresh fruits and vegetables, high-fiber breads, and meats and milk products with no hormones and you can avoid the many negative side effects of processed foods. For more detailed guidance on how to replace the processed foods in your diet with nutritious whole foods, see the recipes in Chapter 17 and the daily meal plans provided in the twenty-one-day plan.

SALT IS PROCESSED TOO

Table salt is processed, heated, and chemically cleaned, plus it contains sodium chloride and chemicals, nothing healthy, and has absolutely nothing in common with natural wholesome salt. Consuming table salt causes excess fluids in your body tissue which can contribute to cellulite, gout, arthritis, rheumatism, and gallstones. The best wholesome, natural salt available today is Himalayan Crystal Salt, and you can find large containers at Whole Foods or a health food store for about seven or eight dollars. It contains all of the eighty-four elements found in your body, and some of its benefits are that it:

- Balances your blood sugar levels and reduces your aging rate.
- Assists in clearing mucus and phlegm from your lungs—helpful for asthma and cystic fibrosis.
- Helps clear up congestion in your sinuses and prevents muscle cramp.
- Regulates your sleeps and maintains your libido.
- Prevents varicose veins and spider veins in your thighs.
- Helps prevent osteoporosis by making the structure of your bones firm.
- Helps regulate your blood pressure.

I know most of you may have never heard of Himalayan Salt but do a little search at your health food store and I am sure you will find this salt, which is recognized as the purest salt on earth. Sea salt would be your next choice, but unfortunately almost 90 percent of all manufacturers are starting to refine sea salt, so be sure to read your labels. Our oceans and seas are also heavily polluted with poisonous toxins, which ultimately affect sea salt.

12

BE CAREFUL WHAT YOU DRINK

When it comes to healthy eating for weight loss and overall wellness, people too often overlook the importance of monitoring what they drink as they focus on what they eat. It is time to put the spotlight on water, soda, juice, alcohol, diet soda, and coffee.

WATER FOR FAT BURNING, WATER FOR HEALING

Your body is already 60 to 70 percent water, but it needs water for just about every biological and chemical process, which means that if you are not getting enough—and three-quarters of us aren't—you are preventing your body from functioning at its best. Unintentional dehydration can lead to all kinds of health problems. When your body needs water, it will scavenge around, looking to draw water from wherever it can. Usually, the first place your body will draw from is the protective lining of your stomach, as well as the walls of your small and large intestines. Depleting your stomach and intestines of water can lead to ulcers and chronic constipation, which in turn can lead to body toxicity as the liver and kidneys are forced to work overtime to keep toxins out of your blood. Proper hydration has been proven to help prevent and/or cure all of the following conditions: constipation, heartburn, stomach ulcers, arthritis, headaches, lower back pain, neck pain, fatigue, asthma, gastrointestinal upset, abdominal pain, acne and other skin diseases, sciatica, allergies, cardiac irregularities, nervousness, high blood pressure, high cholesterol, and Alzheimer's disease.

Water is especially needed in order for fat to burn. The process of fat burning takes place in your muscles at the cellular level, and involves turning the fat you ingest into adenosine triphosphate (ATP), which is your body's basic fuel. Without adequate hydration, the muscle cells cannot function at their best, and you will not be able to transform your ingested fat into usable energy as efficiently, which means more of the fat will stick around to become unwanted flab.

ALCOHOL

You may know that most alcohol is high in calories (7 calories in 1 gram), but you probably don't know the other adverse effects alcohol has on your ability to lose weight. A form of poison, alcohol sends your body into a kind of emergency detoxification mode, as your system tries to neutralize the influx of sugar and toxic chemicals; this means that other processes and functions such as digestion and the utilization of nutrients and energy are interrupted, and your

JEANETTE'S RX

DRINK MORE WATER

Many health experts agree that we should be drinking at least half our body weight in ounces of water a day. (If you weigh 140 pounds, that's 70 ounces of water you should be drinking every single day.)

For convenience, carry water with you all day long—keep a bottle in the car, in your purse, in your gym bag, at your desk, wherever you regularly spend time.

Replace soda and/or juice with water and get the added bonus of reducing calories. The average soda or glass of juice contains 250 to 500 calories, which is the caloric total of a complete, sensible balanced meal. And the quantity of sugar in soda or juice will also send your blood sugar through the roof. You may feel a temporary energy boost but one that will crash quickly and make you crave more sugar.

metabolism slows down. When your body has finished dealing with the sudden inrush of sugar into the blood, you're left with low blood sugar, or hypoglycemia, which gives rise to a false sense of urgent hunger, which in turn gives rise to overeating, and flooding an already compromised metabolism with whatever you can get your hands on. Because alcohol is rapidly absorbed into the small intestine through the stomach, consistent drinking, especially on an empty stomach, can damage the lining of your gastrointestinal tract; combined with many prescription drugs and high stress, consistent drinking can also lead to leaky gut syndrome.

I'm not saying you can never have another cocktail; I know it's unlikely that you're going to quit drinking altogether. Just drink responsibly, and *in moderation*. Try giving your body a break from alcohol for thirty to sixty days and watch that weight melt off. I always make my clients fast from alcohol for at least thirty days. This process builds mental strength and will help you lose more weight. Never drink on an empty stomach—always make sure you consume some protein and fat when you're drinking, to help slow down the absorption of sugar into the bloodstream.

DIET SODA

Another common dieting pitfall is excessive diet soda consumption; most people think that no calories means no problem—they're wrong. Now that you've signed a contract to turn your health around, you have to get into the habit of looking at the ingredients of everything you put into your body; diet soda may be calorie free, but it does have ingredients, and you should know what they are: carbonated water, caramel color, aspartame (NutraSweet) or sucralose (Splenda), phosphoric acid, potassium benzoate, natural flavors, citric acid, caffeine, and phenylketonurics (contains phenylalanine). Sure, carbonated water, natural flavors, and caffeine don't sound so bad. But aspartame has been shown to trigger or worsen the following: brain tumors, migraine headaches, multiple sclerosis, epilepsy, chronic fatigue syndrome, Parkinson's disease, Alzheimer's disease, mental retardation and other birth defects when consumed by pregnant women, lymphoma, fibromyalgia, and diabetes. Sucralose (Splenda) can cause diarrhea, reduced growth rate, decreased red blood cell count, atrophy of lymph follicles in the spleen, enlarged liver and kidneys, and shrunken thymus glands. Studies have also shown artificial sweeteners to stimulate appetite, increase carbohydrate craving, and trigger fat storage and weight gain. So you see, just because they have no calories doesn't mean you won't gain weight from them. Next time you want to reach for a diet soda, choose water instead, and spare your body the chemicals and side effects.

CAFFEINE

I know you were really hoping I wouldn't touch this one because, let's face it, who wants to give up their morning cup of java? But it's important that you understand the side effects of caffeine, which is found not only in coffee but also in dark cola drinks, tea, chocolate, and energy drinks. Caffeine is a diuretic, which means it depletes the body of water and nutrients through urination. So right off the top, for every cup of caffeinated drink that you consume you will need to supply the body with an additional two to three cups of water and then add your daily water intake on top of that.

If you are prone to stress, depression, and anxiety, you will tend to be especially sensitive to the effects of caffeine, which will exacerbate these conditions even further. Caffeine stimulates the release of excess stress hormones (adrenaline) via its stimulating effects on the adrenal glands. It causes the pancreas to secrete insulin, which lowers blood sugar, which in turn forces the body to compensate by releasing stress hormones. These cause the body to release energy, fat, and glucose reserves to stabilize blood sugar levels. Caffeine can exacerbate or even cause stress, anxiety, depression, and insomnia because it interferes with a tranquilizing neurotransmitter chemical in the brain called adenosine. This is the chemical that turns down our anxiety levels—it's our body's version of a tranquilizer. Caffeine docks into a receptor for adenosine and regular use of caffeine is enough to produce anxiety and depression in susceptible individuals. By decreasing or eliminating caffeine you will lower your stress hormone levels and therefore reduce stress, anxiety, and depression. So, the next time you reach for the java, consider some of the great alternatives to caffeinated drinks: naturally decaffeinated coffee, herbal and fruit-flavored teas, and, of course, water.

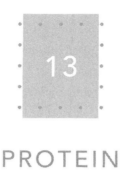

PROTEIN

Protein is the structural material of your body, making up everything from your hair, skin, and nails to your bones, tendons, ligaments, muscles, hormones, and red blood cells.

Protein is also essential to just about every process that goes on within your body, and it gets used up as your body functions from day to day. To ensure that your body is able to synthesize replacement proteins, you need to get the right kinds and combinations of amino acids from your diet. Protein is made up of chains of amino acids, and while there are more than one hundred different kinds of amino acids, there are eight that are particularly important, as they all need to be available in their correct relative amounts for protein synthesis to occur within the body. These are: tryptophan, methionine, valine, threonine, phenylalanine, leucine, isoleucine, and lysine. The best proteins are those that contain the greatest amount and the right percentages of these essential amino acids.

The highest-quality proteins are found in animal products; eggs, raw milk, and most meat proteins are "complete" proteins. That means that they meet all of the body's amino acid requirements for tissue maintenance and growth. Vegetarians and vegans must carefully plan their diets to make sure they get all their essential amino acids and to prevent protein malnutrition. Cereal or grains and legumes (beans and peas) when combined and ingested together provide all the essential amino acids, but in lower quantities, so you have to remain aware of your portion sizes and your caloric guidelines. A bowl of brown rice and beans, for example, will give you your complete proteins, but is also high in calories and carbohydrates. Tofu and soy products are also excellent alternative sources of protein.

It is important to choose protein sources carefully, as some sources are better than others, and some present health risks. Free-range eggs from chickens raised on flaxseeds are going to be healthier than eggs from factory farm chickens that are fed everything from feces to cement filler. Free-range grain-fed beef is better than beef from a cow that's been injected with steroids and hormones, and fed offal. Salmon and tuna are also excellent sources of high-value protein as well as healthy omega-3 fatty acids (I'll cover those in Chapter 14, Fat), but you must be careful of the mercury and other toxins that are found in all fish. (See Chapter 16, Environmental Pollutants, for more information and ways to minimize your risk.) Be a smart consumer: find out where your food comes from, the conditions under which it's been produced, and exactly what's in it. This is especially important when it comes to protein, which your body uses to rebuild your own living cells. You are, quite literally, what you eat.

HOW MUCH PROTEIN DO I NEED?

The Food and Nutrition Board of the Institute of Medicine recommends that you consume 10 to 35 percent of your daily calories from protein, but I, along with many nutritional scientists, recommend that a slightly higher percentage, 25 to 40 percent, of your daily calories coming from protein. What does this mean? Each gram of protein contains 4 calories. Go back to your Calorie Intake and Output charts in Part 2 and look up your daily calorie allowance for food intake to calculate how many grams of protein you should be getting daily. For example, a 30-year-old woman has a daily calorie allowance of 1,575 calories; 25 to 40 percent of that is 394 to 630 calories. Divide both of those numbers by 4, and you have your recommended protein range in grams, 99 to 158.

If you want to get more precise, there are alternative methods of calculating how much protein you need in your diet to achieve your specific weight loss and fitness goals. Research conducted in independent studies suggests that for maximum benefit to developing muscle—and remember, that's *fat-burning* muscle—you should consume roughly 1 gram of protein for every 1 gram of your goal lean body weight. Your lean body weight is simply your regular weight minus the weight of your body fat. For example, Jane Doe, at 5'5", has a regular weight of 140 pounds and a goal body fat of 28 percent; $140 - (140 \times .28) = 100.8$. Jane Doe's goal lean body weight is therefore approximately 101 pounds, so she should be consuming around 100 grams of protein daily.

A TYPICAL DAY'S PROTEIN INTAKE

A 30-year-old woman's daily caloric intake is taken from her Calorie Intake and Output chart: 1,575 calories a day, and with a suggested 100 grams protein daily, this means that 400 calories, or roughly 26 percent of her daily calories, should come from protein. Here's an idea of what this looks like in terms of what you would actually eat in a day:

Breakfast:	2 free-range organic eggs (12.5g protein)
	3 slices turkey bacon (7g protein)
Snack:	½ cup low-fat organic cottage cheese (14g protein)
Lunch:	4 oz. canned tuna (29g protein)
Snack:	¼ cup organic walnuts (4.6g protein)
Snack:	6 ounces plain low-fat yogurt (7.5g protein)
	¼ cup All Bran with extra fiber (1.9g protein)
Dinner:	4 oz. boneless, skinless chicken breast (28.5g protein)
	1 cup broccoli (4.6g protein)
	1 cup carrots (1.7g protein)

Total protein: 111.3g

Total calories from protein: 444

Percentage of daily calories from protein: 28%

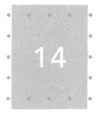

FAT

As we are all painfully aware, our bodies have the ability to turn just about anything we consume into fat. All you have to do is consume more calories in a day than you burn, and the excess will turn into beautiful body fat. In order to lose that body fat, and to maintain good health, you have to know a few things about the fat you are getting from your diet.

There are three different kinds of fat available in the foods we eat: unsaturated fats, which include monounsaturated and polyunsaturated fats and which have been labeled the "good" fats; saturated fats, which have unfairly been labeled the "bad" fats; and trans fats, which are harmful to your body in many ways, and may even cause cancer. The USDA's recommended daily allowance for all fats is 20 to 35 percent of your daily caloric intake. Unfortunately, this general recommendation doesn't take into account the very different effects that various forms of fat have on your body; as a result, Americans in general get too much of the unhealthy processed damaged fat, and not enough of the essential healthy kinds. Let's walk through the three fats so you can start making the right choices when it comes to the fat in your diet.

UNSATURATED FATS

We'll start with the unsaturated good fats. The word *unsaturated* refers to the molecular structure of the fat; unsaturated fatty acids (which is just the biological term for unsaturated fats) are more liquid than saturated fatty acids, and do not form solids easily. Unsaturated fat tends to disperse itself and is antisticky, so the molecules move around apart from each other. All of these properties make unsaturated fatty acids fluid and flexible, which means they are able to move freely within the body, making and breaking contacts with one another to fulfill important chemical and transport functions. This fluidity also means that unsaturated fatty acids do not form clots in the bloodstream.

Within the unsaturated fat family, there are two groups differentiated by their molecular makeup: monounsaturated fatty acids, which contain one double bond, and polyunsaturated fatty acids, which contain more than one double bond.

MONOUNSATURATED FATS

Unlike polyunsaturated fats, monounsaturated fats are produced naturally in the body from other fats, and for that reason are considered nonessential fatty acids. Many kinds exist, but there are currently two that are well known for their nutritional importance. Palmitoleic acid is found in animal fats, milk, and macadamia nuts as well as in unrefined coconut and palm oils. Palmitoleic acid is an antimicrobial fat that protects us against pathogens in the gut, functions as an emulsifying agent in biological systems, and is particularly involved in the transportation of fats within the body. Oleic acid is found in olive, almond, peanut, pistachio, pecan, canola, avocado, hazelnut, cashew, and macadamia oils, as well as in the fat deposits of most land animals; its main function is to keep our arteries supple.

Although both of these monounsaturated fatty acids are considered beneficial, in excess they can interfere with the body's ability to produce prostaglandins, important hormone-like substances that regulate a range of cell functions on a moment-to-moment basis. Prostaglandins modify the muscle tone of our blood vessels, lower blood pressure, relax coronary arteries, and inhibit platelet stickiness; other prostaglandins have exact countereffects within the body, and it's the delicate balance between these opposing functions that keeps your cardiovascular system, as well as other systems, in healthy working order.

POLYUNSATURATED FATS: THE ESSENTIAL FATS

Unlike monounsaturated fats, all-important polyunsaturated fats are not produced within the body naturally, and therefore must be imported to the body via your food. The two most important polyunsaturated fatty acids are linoleic acid (LA), an omega-6 fatty acid, and alpha-linoleic acid (LNA), an omega-3 fatty acid: these are known variously as the essential fats, the essential fatty acids, and the essential oils, and are absolutely integral to the ongoing healthy function of your body.

Essential fatty acids, or EFAs, feed every part of us, providing energy-rich fuel to every cell, tissue, gland, and organ; they are also integral to all body structures and many bodily functions. Throughout our lifetime our brains, nerves, hearts, arteries, and reproductive systems need and use essential fats. Essential fatty acids are densest and most needed in our brains and nervous systems, which is why as humans, we need more fat than any other creature on the planet.

LINOLEIC ACID (LA) OMEGA-6 FATTY ACID

Linoleic acid is most abundant in safflower and sunflower oils, but is also found in corn, sesame, hemp, soybean, walnut, pumpkin seed, flaxseed, cottonseed, almond, rice bran, and olive oils. The average American diet contains plenty of linoleic acid, so deficiency in this fat is not something you need to worry about. Symptoms of a deficiency include eczema-like skin eruptions, hair loss, water loss through the skin with attendant thirst, behavioral changes, fatty infiltration of the liver, kidney malfunction, drying up of the glands, susceptibility to infection, failure to heal wounds, sterility in males, miscarriage in females, arthritis-like conditions, heart arrhythmia, growth retardation, dry skin and eyes, brittle nails and hair, and elevated cholesterol.

ALPHA-LINOLENIC ACID (LNA) OMEGA-3 FATTY ACID

Alpha-linolenic acid is found most abundantly in flaxseed oil, the fat content of which is more than 50 percent LNA; it is also found in oils from chia and kukui (30 percent LNA), hemp seed (20 percent LNA), pumpkin seed (15 percent LNA), canola (up to 10 percent LNA), walnuts (3 to 11 percent LNA), and soybeans (5 to 7 percent LNA), as well as in wheat germ and dark green leafy vegetables in lesser quantities.

Unlike its essential fatty acid counterpart, LNA is seriously lacking in our traditional Western diets. Some symptoms of omega-3 deficiency include growth retardation, behavioral changes, weakness, diminished vision, learning problems, depression, hyperactivity, attention deficit, dyslexia, poor motor coordination, poor muscle growth, impaired ability to heal from injuries, tingling sensation in the limbs and extremities, insulin resistance, high cholesterol, high blood pressure, tendency to form arterial clots, tissue inflammation, leaky gut, allergies, autoimmune conditions, increased susceptibility to tumor growth, water retention and swelling, dry or inflamed skin, low metabolism, low energy, lower thyroid and adrenal function, and in males, low testosterone levels. As you can see, not getting enough LNA in your diet lays the ground for some serious health problems.

FISH OILS

In addition to the two essentials LA omega-6 and LNA omega-3, there are two more omega-3 fatty acids that provide amazing health benefits. Eicosapentaenoic acid (EPA) and docosahexaenoic acid (DHA) can be produced in the body and so are technically considered nonessential; but the body can only produce EPA and DHA from the essential fat LNA, and since most Americans suffer from an LNA deficiency, their ability to produce EPA and DHA is compromised. EPA and DHA can be found in salmon, trout, mackerel, sardines, Alaskan halibut, herring, sea bass, oysters, clams, and eel. Fish oil supplements can also be taken to get your daily dose of these two wonderful fats.

Both EPA and DHA are especially abundant in the most biochemically active tissues in our body, namely the brain cells, nerve relay stations (synapses), visual receptors (retina), adrenal glands, and sex glands. They are the most unsaturated of all the fats, and their tendency to disperse and move apart from one another is so strong that they can prevent aggregation of the saturated fatty acids that like to stick together to form blood clots and arterial blockages.

EPA and DHA are metabolized by the body very slowly: it takes about two weeks for us to completely break these fats down, and this is roughly how long their extraordinarily beneficial effects last within our bodies. To maintain these protective effects, you should eat fish at least every two weeks. The fish should not be fried; sushi and sashimi are excellent sources of EPA and DHA, and the best way to cook your fish is to broil it whole. High-fat, cold-water fish is best eaten with its skin on, as the oils we want are found there.

HOW MUCH ESSENTIAL FAT DO I NEED?

Research and national governing bodies vary in their recommendations for the amount of essential fat you need in your diet for optimum health. You should note that the following guidelines are for healthy adults; if you suffer from coronary heart disease or from high cholesterol levels, you should obtain your requirements from your doctor. The Food and Nutrition Board of the Institute of Medicine recommends that you get 5 to 10 percent of your daily calories from LA omega-6 fatty acids, or approximately 11 to 12 grams for women or 16 to 17 grams for men. It encourages getting these fats from nuts, seeds, and soybean, safflower, and corn oils. For LNA omega-3 fatty acids, it recommends a daily percentage of 0.6 to 1.2 percent, or approximately 1.1 grams for women and 1.6 grams for men; that you get these fats from fish oils, fatty fish, and oils such as canola, soybean, and flaxseed; and that you get very little of these fats from eggs and meat.

The American Heart Association suggests eating a variety of (preferably fatty) fish at least twice a week and to incorporate oils and foods rich in LNA omega-3, such as flaxseed, canola, and soybean oils, and walnuts.

Dr. Udo Erasmus, Ph.D., who has studied fats and their effects on our health for more than twenty years and is considered one of the world's leading authorities on the subject, has slightly higher recommendations. He advocates getting between 3 and 6 percent of your daily calories from LA omega-6 fatty acids, or approximately 9 to 18 grams, about one tablespoon, per day. For LNA omega-3 fatty acids, he supports a daily percentage of 2 percent, or between 2 and 9 grams, which is about one or two teaspoons a day.

The percentages of your daily calorie intake from each authority are very close, so I recommend a range that falls within both recommendations: 3 to 10 percent of your daily calories from omega-6 fatty acids and 1.5 to 2 percent of your daily calories from omega-3 fatty acids.

When you start adding essential fats to your diet, make sure that you are also getting healthy amounts of vitamins C, B_3, and B_6, as well as the minerals magnesium and zinc; these must all be present in your body in order for it to be able to metabolize the essential fats. A multivitamin and balanced meal plan will take care of these requirements, and you won't have to worry that you're missing out on any of the wonderful benefits of essential fats.

The other thing to be aware of as you begin to incorporate the essential fats into your life is that the sources you choose should be unrefined and as pure as possible. To maximize shelf life manufacturers often treat oils with refining, degumming, bleaching, and deodorizing agents, which damage the essential fat content and reduce the health benefits. Essential oils should be cold pressed from organically grown seeds and nuts. As they are very chemically sensitive and easily damaged by light, air, and heat, they are best stored in brown glass and refrigerated.

All the oils I have mentioned above can be bought in most health food stores and through Internet suppliers. Some of them are also getting picked up by major supermarket chains, which is a great sign that more and more people are seeking out the best for their bodies and their lives. It's time for you to join them!

I have touched upon the important biological functions of the essential fatty acids, but now that you are familiar with your omega-6 and your omega-3, let's get specific about how they will help you reach your goals. There are so many benefits you will derive from upping your essential fat intake that it would take pages and pages to list them all, but here are some important ones for anyone who is trying to lose weight and get healthy.

Essential fats will help you toward your weight-loss goals in all of the following ways:

1. Essential fats shuttle oxygen to the cells in your body, where it is needed to burn fat, thus increasing fat-burning activity and in turn boosting your energy levels, motivating you toward more physical activity, and resulting in additional calorie burning.

2. Essential fats support greater metabolic function by helping your body make greater use of its stores of body fat for energy.

3. By increasing insulin efficiency, essential fats help to ensure that you don't develop excess insulin in the blood, a condition that will signal your body to slow down its fat-burning activities and that triggers fat storage.

4. Essential fats increase activity in several genes that make enzymes for fat burning, while decreasing the activity of several other genes that make enzymes for fat and storage.

5. Not getting the vital nutrients in essential fats renders you more susceptible to cravings for junk food, starches, and sweets; obtaining the missing essential fats will satisfy the cravings without your having to make unwise food choices.

6. Essential fats reduce the time required for your muscles to recover from fatigue after working out by facilitating the conversion of lactic acid (the substance produced in your muscles during exercise) into water and carbon dioxide.

7. Essential fats support and facilitate increased production of serotonin, a neurotransmitter that helps to decrease stress and anxiety, and lift depression.

Quite aside from the benefits associated with weight loss, essential fats also help support your total health for years to come. Here are a few of the long-term health benefits:

1. Essential fats, specifically EPA and DHA (found in fish oil supplements and cold-water fish), work to keep your blood from getting too sticky, which decreases the

likelihood of clots that can lead to heart attack and stroke. EPA also supports production of hormone-like prostaglandins, which helps reduce the risk of clotting and problems that may arise from clotting such as cardiovascular complications accompanying diabetes. Prostaglandins also help to keep the heartbeat regular, preventing arrhythmia that could lead to cardiac arrest, and they lower excessively high levels of lipoprotein, a very strong risk factor for heart and artery disease.

2. Essential fats lower blood pressure by producing the kinds of prostaglandins that decrease blood pressure and block the production of blood pressure–raising agents. Essential fats also lower blood pressure by relaxing arterial muscle tone.

3. Essential fats reduce your risk of cancer and other immune system diseases. Studies have shown that omega-3 and omega-6 fatty acids from plant and fish oils not only inhibit the growth of tumors but also protect you at the cellular level against toxins by sacrificing themselves to harmful substances that would otherwise damage vital cell structures. Essential fats also carry toxins out of your body through the skin, which helps lighten the work of your liver and kidneys, which might otherwise become poisoned.

4. Essential fats reduce high cholesterol, lowering excessive triglycerides by up to 65 percent—which is better than any drug—and increasing good HDL cholesterol. The nutrients found in organic, unrefined essential oils also block cholesterol absorption and reabsorption into the gut. All in all they can lower your total cholesterol count by up to 25 percent.

5. Essential fats aid and improve our digestive systems, acting as anti-inflammatory agents within the stomach and improving gut integrity, which helps prevent leaky gut and food allergies. They protect beneficial gut bacteria, and encourage the growth of beneficial bowel flora. And by reducing loss of water through the skin, they make it unnecessary for the body to pull water from the bowel, protecting against constipation and the toxic consequences of colon dehydration.

6. Essential fats improve all areas of brain function. Not only do they promote the production of serotonin, which decreases anxiety and lifts depression, but they also improve your mental processing, learning skills, visual acuity, and color perception. Further research has also indicated a connection between omega-3 fats and decreased risk of hyperactivity disorders, Alzheimer's disease, bipolar disease, schizophrenia, dementia, and clinical depression.

7. For the women out there, essential fats can ease, and often completely reverse, premenstrual syndrome.

As you can see, the benefits to your health are many as well as invaluable. Get the essential fats into your diet, and your body will thank you inside, outside, and for years to come!

SATURATED FATS

Saturated fats have been labeled unfairly by leading health organizations and conventional medical experts as the unhealthy counterpart to the "good fats" discussed above. It is important to note that there are two schools of thought on the benefits and risks of saturated fats. Both are represented by intelligent and qualified doctors, nutritionists, and researchers. One school is composed of medical experts who believe and follow conventional medicine, the other is composed of medical experts who believe in homeopathic and alternative medicine.

The conventional medical experts, pharmaceutical companies, leading health organizations, and manufacturers of refined vegetable oils espouse the belief that saturated fats are the bad fats that cause high cholesterol and heart disease. They support their claims with the "lipid theory," which posits that a diet high in cholesterol and saturated fat will cause "gooey" substances (cholesterols) to be deposited in the blood vessels. Clogged blood vessels clearly restrict blood flow to the heart, ultimately causing angina. Eventually a piece or "clot" will break loose, causing a transient ischemic attack (TIA: angina or a ministroke), a stroke, or a full-blown heart attack.

The holistic and alternative medical experts hold that before the 1920s (the beginning of the launch of refined and processed foods) heart disease was rare in America and that saturated fats are not the cause of our modern diseases. They believe that the scientific evidence, honestly evaluated, does not support the assertion that "artery-clogging" saturated fats cause heart disease. Actually, evaluation of the fat in clogged arteries reveals that only about 26 percent is saturated. The rest is unsaturated, of which more than half is polyunsaturated. Holistic and alternative medical experts believe that heart disease, cancer, immune system dysfunction, sterility, learning disabilities, growth problems, and osteoporosis are caused by the processed foods and processed oils that have been added to the American diet since the 1920s; that is, all hydrogenated oils, soy, corn, and safflower oils, cottonseed oil, canola oil, and all other fats that are heated to very high temperatures during processing and cooking.

THE REAL KILLERS

Conventional food manufacturers, governing bodies, doctors, and researchers have been claiming saturated fat and cholesterol as the heart disease killers for more than twenty years, but with all of the cholesterol-lowering pharmaceutical drugs and cholesterol-free and fat-free products available today, heart disease is still the number one killer in America. Don't be fooled; processed foods and large portion sizes are to blame.

The holistic and alternative medical experts further outline the importance of healthy saturated fats in our bodies. Healthy saturated fats:

- constitute at least 50 percent of the cell membranes.
- play a vital role in the health of our bones. For calcium to be effectively incorporated into the skeletal structure, at least 50 percent of the dietary fats must be saturated.
- lower a substance in the blood that indicates proneness to heart disease. They protect the liver from alcohol and other toxins, such as Tylenol.
- enhance the immune system.
- are needed for the proper utilization of essential fatty acids. Elongated omega-3 fatty acids are better retained in the tissues when the diet is rich in saturated fats.
- are the preferred foods for the heart, which is why the fat around the heart muscle is highly saturated. The heart draws on this reserve of fat in times of stress.
- have important antimicrobial properties. They protect us against harmful microorganisms in the digestive tract.

Healthy saturated fats are fats that are not processed or refined, that are nutrient rich, and that occur naturally. Examples of healthy saturated fats are unrefined organic coconut oil, palm oil, sesame oil, cold pressed olive oil, cold pressed flaxseed oil, organic raw milk, organic butter, fish oils, and organic animal fat found in organic meat.

The American Heart Association, which supports the "lipid theory," recommends limiting saturated fat intake to 10 percent or less of your daily calories for healthy people, and less than 7 percent for anyone with coronary heart disease, diabetes, or high cholesterol. Saturated fats are found in all food fats and oils and in large quantities in animal fats (red meat, lamb, pork, duck, butter fat, milk fat), lard (deep-fried foods), and coconut and palm oils.

Personally, I favor the holistic and alternative medical perspective on saturated fats. I recommend that 7 to 20 percent of your daily calories should come from high-quality healthy saturated fat such as unprocessed organic animal foods: meat, fish, free-range eggs, organic or raw milk products; and unprocessed organic saturated fats, including olive oil, butter, peanut oil, palm oil, coconut oil, and animal fats.

TRANS FATS

There are many different kinds of trans fat that can be found in many different places, including in small amounts naturally occurring in plants and animals; but there's one kind that is particularly dangerous for your health, and it's the kind that is especially prevalent in the American diet, the kind that is produced when a normal unsaturated fat or oil is chemically altered in a process called hydrogenation.

Hydrogenation is the process whereby unsaturated fats are acted upon so that their molecular structure is changed to give them longer shelf lives in baked products, to provide longer fry life for cooking oils, and to produce a certain kind of texture or "mouth feel." Hydrogenation is bad not only because it chemically alters the essential fatty acids present in the original natural oil, but also because the process involves the use of toxic metals, traces of which remain with the fat when it is consumed by us. Particularly worrisome is the use of aluminum, which in the human body has been linked to Alzheimer's disease and osteoporosis, and may even speed the development of cancer. Trans fats are created when the process of hydrogenation has not been completed, which is called partial hydrogenation; this is the process used to make margarine, shortening, shortening oil, and partially hydrogenated vegetable oil. These products, heavily used in chain fast-food restaurants (to make french fries, onion rings, and doughnuts) and packaged goods (cookies, cakes, crackers, and chips) contain large quantities of deadly trans fats.

Trans fats have been shown to increase bad LDL cholesterol and decrease good HDL cholesterol. They have been shown to interfere with our liver's detoxification system, and with essential fatty acid function within the body. They have also been linked to an increased risk of cancer.

In addition to partially hydrogenated fats, food manufacturers will use completely hydrogenated fats to increase shelf life; although these have been shown to raise bad cholesterol and contain unnatural fatty acid molecules and other particles that may be toxic, they do not contain any trans fats like their partially hydrogenated counterparts.

I recommend that you really try to avoid trans fats as much as possible; instead choose wholesome foods with naturally forming, undamaged healthy fats rather than products that are deep fried or highly processed.

Tracking the exact percentages of the different types of fat consumed in your diet is next to impossible because food manufacturers only label the amount of TOTAL fat, saturated fat, and cholesterol. Remember, conventional food manufacturers are part of the school that believes and supports "the lipid theory"; therefore they believe the only numbers that are important to you are the numbers indicating the amount of saturated fat and cholesterol. Over several years the holistic and alternative medical experts have pressured the FDA to require manufacturers to list the amount of dangerous trans fats on food labels and finally, as of 2006, it is now mandatory. To get your daily dose of healthy fats, just make sure that three to six meals include at least one food item that contains wholesome, high-quality, unprocessed, unrefined fat. Staying within your daily total caloric allowance is also important, so portion control is necessary.

JEANETTE'S RX

DAILY RECOMMENDATIONS FOR FAT INTAKE
20–35 percent of daily calories from all fats
7–20 percent of daily calories from unprocessed healthy saturated fats
3–10 percent of your daily calories from omega-6 fatty acids
1.5–2 percent of your daily calories from omega-3 fatty acids

A TYPICAL DAY'S FAT INTAKE

Here is what a typical daily intake should look like for a thirty-year-old woman with a daily caloric allowance of 1,575 calories. (There are 9 calories in 1 gram of fat.)

Breakfast:	2 free-range organic eggs (8g fat)
	3 slices turkey bacon (5g fat) (Applegate Farms makes delicious organic turkey bacon.)
Snack:	½ cup organic low-fat cottage cheese (2g fat)
Lunch:	4 oz. canned tuna (1g fat)
Snack:	¼ cup organic walnuts (17g fat)
Snack:	6 oz. plain low-fat yogurt (2g fat)
Dinner:	4 oz. boneless, skinless organic chicken breast (2g fat)
	½ tablespoon organic olive oil (7g fat)
Dessert:	2 low-fat oatmeal cookies (5g fat)

Nutritional Supplement: 1 tablespoon organic cold-pressed flaxseed oil, cod liver oil, or fish oil supplement

Total fat: 49g fat

Total calories from protein: 455

Percentage of daily calories from fat: 29%

15

CARBOHYDRATES

The recent low-carb-diet craze has left many people with the impression that carbs are the enemy. This is absolutely not true. Carbohydrates are essential to your diet, providing fuel for your muscles and important nutrients for your brain. There are two kinds of carbohydrates that occur naturally in our food: simple sugars and complex carbohydrates, also known as starches. Simple sugars are found in honey, sugar, milk, and some sweet ripe fruits like grapes, apples, and tomatoes. Complex carbs, or starches, occur in grains, breads, cereals, pastas, vegetables, legumes such as peas and beans, and rice. Both kinds are necessary to a healthy functioning body.

So when it comes to carbs, it's not a matter of cutting them out entirely, as many of the recent diet fads would have you believe—it's a matter of choosing the right kinds. The single biggest problem with the American diet is also the single biggest problem with our carbohydrate consumption: we are choosing processed carbs, which are poor in nutrients and high in sugar, salt, and calories that do not nourish our bodies. Such carbs have lost most, if not all, of their nutritional value, and are chock-full of unnatural chemical preservatives that prolong shelf life but harm your body. Examples of carbs to avoid include white bread, white pasta, white rice, cookies, cakes, deep-fried foods, fruit drinks, sodas, conventional and processed milk products, fried potato/corn chips, candies, and all types of junk food.

Instead, get your carbs from fresh fruits and vegetables, whole wheat bread, whole wheat pasta, brown rice, nuts, beans, high-fiber cereals and snacks, brown-rice cakes, and organic or raw milk products.

HOW MANY CARBS DO I NEED?

Wholesome, unprocessed carbs should make up 30 to 60 percent of your daily caloric intake. The range is relatively wide because different people do well with different amounts of carbs in their diet. For some, a 60 percent carb intake is too high and leads to sluggishness and low energy; for others, a 30 percent carb intake is too low, which leads to the same kinds of fatigue. You

A TYPICAL DAY'S CARB INTAKE

A 30-year-old woman with a daily allowance of 1,575 calories and a range of 30 to 60 percent of calories (472 to 945 calories) from carbs (there are 4 calories in 1 gram of carbohydrate) might follow a daily meal plan that includes:

Breakfast:	1 slice Ezekiel Bread (18g carbs)
Snack:	½ cup blueberries (10g carbs)
Lunch:	1 whole wheat pita (30g carbs)
Snack:	¼ cup organic walnuts (4g carbs)
	2 tablespoons dried cranberries (24g carbs)
Snack:	¼ cup All Bran with extra fiber (11g carbs)
Dinner:	1 cup steamed broccoli (8g carbs)
	1 cup steamed baby carrots (16g carbs)
Dessert:	2 low-fat oatmeal cookies (18g carbs)

Total carbs: 139 grams
Total calories from carbs: 556
Percentage of calories from carbs: 35%

can figure out where within the range you fall by paying attention to your body and adjusting your carb intake levels according to what makes you feel and function the best. You can't go wrong as long as you are choosing wholesome, nutrient-rich carbs that have not been processed or otherwise chemically altered and you are staying within your daily caloric allowance.

INSULIN, GLUCAGON, AND FAT LOSS

Get your carbs in balanced meals that contain the right proportions of carbs (30 to 60 percent), proteins (25 to 40 percent), and essential fats (20 to 35 percent). When you eat meals that are imbalanced and contain large amounts of carbs, you are essentially dumping a whole lot of sugar into your bloodstream at once, with no protein or fat to act as a buffer between the sugar and your blood; this triggers a sudden release of insulin, which in turn causes your body to try to hold on to its fat rather than use it for energy. Conversely, when you eat meals that contain the right proportions of wholesome high-fiber carbs, essential fats, and quality protein, your pancreas will release glucagon, which causes fat burning and helps regulate blood sugar levels. The daily meal plans included in Part 3 give you three weeks' worth of healthy, balanced menus, getting you into the habit of eating right so that you can keep up the good work long after the twenty-one-day plan is over.

FIBER

When choosing your sources of carbohydrates, it is important to look for ones that are high in fiber. Fiber slows the absorption of sugar into the blood, helps eliminate bile acids and cholesterol, and promotes healthy bowel function, so you need to make sure your body has enough. Grains like cereals, crackers, breads, rice, flour, and pasta must have at least 5 grams of fiber per serving to do you any good. Fiber is highest in carbs that are unprocessed and unrefined—yet another reason to avoid "manufactured" foods. The Food and Nutrition Board of the Institute of Medicine recommends that adult women consume 25 grams of fiber a day, and adult men 38 grams. Dr. Steven Pratt, author of the wonderful *SuperFood Rx* books, urges slightly higher daily fiber intakes, 32 grams for women and 45 grams for men. My recommendation is that you hit it somewhere between the two; for women, a daily intake of 25 to 32 grams is ideal, and for men anything from 38 to 45 grams is great.

Some excellent sources of fiber include kidney beans, lima beans, peas, split peas, lentils, Brussels sprouts, broccoli, Swiss chard, chickpeas (found in hummus), black beans, black-eyed peas, corn, popcorn, spinach, zucchini, potato with skin, yam, parsnip, asparagus, prunes, apples, applesauce, bananas, pears, raisins, kiwifruit, oranges, strawberries, almonds, whole grain cereals, brown rice, buckwheat pancakes, barley, flaxseed, soy nuts, wheat germ, whole grain breads, whole wheat flour, and Ezekiel bread (no flour).

A TYPICAL DAY'S FIBER INTAKE

The daily meal plan provided in the carbs section also serves as an example of a day that would include an ample amount of fiber. Here is the breakdown of individual fiber content:

Breakfast:	1 slice Ezekiel Bread (5g fiber)
Snack:	½ cup blueberries (2g fiber)
Lunch:	1 whole wheat pita (5g fiber)
Snack:	¼ cup organic walnuts (4g fiber)
	2 tablespoons dried cranberries (5g fiber)
Snack:	¼ cup All Bran with extra fiber (8g fiber)
Dinner:	1 cup steamed broccoli (5g fiber)
	1 cup steamed baby carrots (5g fiber)
Dessert:	2 low-fat oatmeal cookies (2g fiber)

Total fiber: 41 grams

16

ENVIRONMENTAL POLLUTANTS

Chemical pesticides and environmental pollutants such as mercury and benzene dioxins have found their way into our air, soil, rivers, lakes, and oceans. Many of these toxins end up deposited in the fatty tissue of the fish living in the contaminated water, and are known to damage the nervous, respiratory, and digestive systems; impair reproductive, liver, and brain function; and increase the risk of cancer. Poisoning from consuming mercury in fish has been given the most attention in recent years. In order to decrease your vulnerability to mercury and other ghastly toxins, limit your fish intake to three or four meals a week, and take a week off every now and then; eating a few fish meals a week probably presents little or negligible human health risks. Shark, swordfish, king mackerel, and tilefish contain high levels of mercury, while salmon, catfish, and tuna contain low levels. Canned albacore tuna contains more mercury than canned light tuna. Avoid eating the internal organs of fish, which have a high toxin content. When you prepare most kinds of fish, remove the skin, dark muscle tissue, and any fat you can. Because the healthy omega-3 fatty acids are located in the fat and close to the skin you are removing, you may want to consider taking a fish oil supplement from a highly recommended brand like Carlson's. Being forced to use these kinds of substitutes to obtain beneficial nutrients is the price we pay for continuing to pollute our natural resources. Choose smaller, younger fish, as these generally contain lower levels of contaminants than larger, older fish. In addition, make sure you are eating fish from a variety of bodies of water, which reduces your risk of exposure to any one group of toxic contaminants.

Please be aware that children and women who are nursing, pregnant, or preparing for pregnancy should follow these guidelines provided by the Food and Drug Administration (FDA) and the Environmental Protection Agency (EPA):

1. Avoid shark, swordfish, king mackerel, and tilefish because they contain high levels of mercury.

2. Eat up to twelve ounces (two average meals) a week of a variety of fish and shellfish that are lower in mercury.

   a. Five of the most commonly eaten fish and shellfish that are low in mercury are shrimp, canned light tuna, salmon, pollock, and catfish.

   b. Another commonly eaten fish, albacore ("white") tuna, has more mercury than canned light tuna. So, when choosing your two meals of fish and shellfish, you may eat up to six ounces (one average meal) of albacore tuna per week.

3. Check local advisories about the safety of fish caught by family and friends in your local lakes, rivers, and coastal areas. If no advice is available, eat up to six ounces (one average meal) per week of fish you catch from local waters, but don't consume any other fish during that week.

It pays to conserve our planet by limiting the amount of toxins released into the environment, which eventually end up right back in your food and in your body. Then you have to deal with the side effects, just as the plants, animals, air, and bodies of water do. Remember that saving the environment will also help save your health. We are dependent on Mother Nature for survival, so let's take care of her! Here is a list of seven things you can do to help:

1. Bike, walk, carpool, or take public transportation whenever possible instead of driving.
2. Buy a fuel-efficient or electric vehicle.
3. Drink your morning tea or coffee from a reusable cup and water from a reusable bottle.
4. Recycle all of your paper, plastics, glass, and cans.
5. Use environmentally friendly household cleaning products.

6. Support restaurants and stores that carry recyclable containers, environmentally friendly products, and organic food.

7. Turn off your lights, computers, televisions, and home appliances when you are not using them.

For more information on environmental pollutants, go to www.epa.gov.

There's a lot of information about nutrition in this part of the book, so you'll probably come back from time to time for a refresher, but there will be reminders of key points every day of the twenty-one-day program laid out in Part 5. For those of you who want to know more—because this is really just the tip of the iceberg—I've included a list of recommended reading in Part 6. You can also visit my Web site at www.thehollywoodtrainer.com. If there's one message I want to leave you with on the subject of nutrition, it's that you must start being aware of what you eat. When you're grocery shopping, read labels and apply the knowledge provided here. Try to shop at organic grocery stores like Wild Oats or Whole Foods. They are your best bet but there's also a lot of organic food being offered at supermarkets nowadays, mostly in response to the growing demand. Get into the habit of making wise food choices: seek out items that are wholesome, high in fiber (at least 3 to 5 grams per serving) and essential fats (omega-6, omega-3), and low in sugar (less than 13 grams per serving). Look for lean cuts of meat and—I cannot stress this enough—avoid processed, refined foods in favor of edibles that are as close as possible to their natural whole state. Always remember, you are what you eat. A new life starts on the inside, and now that you have the facts—and the wisdom—you need, you're on your way!

17

THE RECIPES

There is something for everyone—even the pickiest eater or the most inexperienced cook—in these eighty-two wholesome, healthy, and mouthwatering recipes. Don't be afraid to try something new, because you don't want to miss out on a terrific meal.

I haven't used any fat-free, sugar-free, or carb-free products—just wholesome, nutritious ingredients that your body needs in healthy proportions. When you are finished with a meal you will feel happy and satisfied. Remember, whenever possible, to choose organic foods or produce from your local farmers for your meals, because you are literally what you eat!

BERRY BANANA OATMEAL

Oatmeal fits into everyone's budget, is inexpensive, and is good for you. Its fiber slows down the rate of emptying in the stomach, making you feel fuller longer. Oatmeal helps reduce cholesterol levels and is an excellent source of dietary fiber, vitamin E, zinc, selenium, copper, iron, manganese, and magnesium. Choose organic wholesome oats, when possible. You can vary the toppings of fresh fruit and nuts according to your own preferences. *1 serving*

1 cup water
½ cup rolled oats
½ cup blueberries

¼ cup dried cranberries
½ banana, sliced
½ cup organic low-fat milk

In a heavy saucepan, bring water to a full rolling boil. Gradually add the oats, stirring constantly. Turn the heat to low and cook, uncovered, stirring often, until no raw taste remains, or according to the package instructions. Depending on the kind of oats you use, cooking times will vary from 5 minutes (for rolled oats) to 20 minutes or longer (for steel-cut oats). Serve topped with blueberries, cranberries, banana, and milk.

NUTRITIONAL INFORMATION PER SERVING:
429 calories · 10g protein · 92g carbohydrates · 10g fiber · 4g fat · 0mg sodium

MUSCLE OATS

A little protein pump for your morning oats! Adding a scoop of protein powder to your oatmeal is a great way to boost the breakfast of champions. Oatmeal is an amazing breakfast that gives you sustained energy. It has virtually no sodium, sugar, or cholesterol, so it is an excellent breakfast for just about everyone. You can use your favorite whey or soy protein powder. Make sure you read the ingredients because it is a processed food and you definitely want to avoid chemical additives and artificial sweeteners. Designer Whey is one of the most popular brands of protein powder available at most health food stores and supermarkets. You can get organic whey protein powders from such sources as Source Naturals, Frontier, Whey Healthier, Don Lemmon's Complete Protein Powder, and Warrior Milk. *1 serving*

1 cup water
½ cup rolled oats
2 scoops Designer Whey vanilla protein powder
½ cup sliced strawberries
1 ounce walnuts (about 14 halves)

In a heavy saucepan, bring water to a full rolling boil. Gradually add the oats, stirring constantly. Turn the heat to low and cook, uncovered, stirring often, until no raw taste remains, or according to the package instructions. Depending on the kind of oats you use, cooking times will vary from 5 minutes (for rolled oats) to 20 minutes or longer (for steel-cut oats). Add the protein powder to the warm oatmeal and stir until all of the whey has dissolved. Top with strawberries and walnuts. If you prefer to have your oatmeal with milk, you can add ½ cup organic low-fat milk but you will have to add the additional calories to your nutritional counts (see chart, pp. 246–254).

NUTRITIONAL INFORMATION PER SERVING:
395 calories · 31g protein · 51g carbohydrates · 8g fiber · 9g fat · 1mg sodium

FAST-AND-EASY POACHED EGGS

Over the years I have encountered many people who find it difficult and time-consuming to make poached eggs. I love them because they're smooth and delicious, and they can never burn in the pan. Try to use organic eggs from farm-raised chickens that have been fed on flaxseed since the yolks contain healthy fat. *1 serving*

2 large eggs
Freshly ground black pepper, to taste

Pour about 2 inches of water into a shallow saucepan or skillet (not iron). Bring to a gentle boil and adjust the heat so water simmers. Break the eggs one at a time into a small bowl, and then add carefully in the simmering water. (If you swirl the water into a whirlpool as you are adding the eggs they will hold together better.) Sprinkle with ground pepper. Cook for 2 to 5 minutes, checking for doneness to your taste. If you like your yolks soft or medium, remove them as soon as all of the white is fully cooked. Remove with a slotted spoon and serve.

NUTRITIONAL INFORMATION PER SERVING:

148 calories · 12g protein · 1g carbohydrates · 10g fat · 3g saturated fat · 126mg sodium · 0g fiber

CHEF STEPHANIE'S FRITTATA

Chef Stephanie is well-known in Hollywood among A-list celebrities for bringing a gourmet touch to healthy dishes. The prosciutto di Parma may seem expensive but even a very small amount gives a lot of flavor and is much better than bacon or other cured meat. *1 serving*

¾ cup egg whites (from approximately 6 large egg whites)
2 tablespoons half-and-half
Butter-flavored cooking spray
1 teaspoon minced shallots
2 tablespoons finely chopped prosciutto di Parma

1 tablespoon finely diced red potato
1 medium Roma tomato, finely diced
1 teaspoon grated Parmesan cheese
3 fresh basil leaves, cut into very thin strips (chiffonade)
Freshly ground black pepper, to taste

Preheat the broiler. In a medium bowl, beat the egg whites and half-and-half until frothy. Coat a small, ovenproof skillet with butter-flavored cooking spray. Sauté the shallots over medium heat until fragrant, then add the prosciutto and cook for about 3 minutes, or until the prosciutto starts to crisp. Add the diced potato and cook for 3 more minutes, then add the tomato and cook for 1 more minute. Turn down the heat to medium-low, pour the egg white mixture evenly over the vegetables, and cook without stirring until the mixture starts to firm up. Top with the Parmesan cheese and half of the basil and place under the heated broiler on the top rack or 4 to

5 inches from the heat source and cook for about 6 minutes, or until frittata is lightly browned. Remove from broiler, turn out onto a heated plate, and top with the remaining fresh basil and ground pepper to taste.

NUTRITIONAL INFORMATION PER SERVING:

224 calories · 29g protein · 10g carbohydrates · 6g fat · 3g saturated fat · 1,065mg sodium · 0g fiber

OATMEAL–EGG WHITE BREAKFAST FRITTATA

This is a good healthy alternative to pancakes, and one of my personal favorites. Using oatmeal instead of refined flour makes this dish higher in fiber and more nutritious than pancakes.

1 serving

3 large egg whites
¼ cup rolled oats
½ tablespoon olive oil
½ cup low-sodium organic low-fat
    cottage cheese

½ cup sliced strawberries
½ cup sliced banana
¼ cup applesauce

In a small bowl, mix the egg whites and oats until combined. Heat the olive oil in a heavy small skillet over medium heat. Pour the oatmeal mixture into the warm pan and cook without stirring for 3 to 4 minutes, until browned underneath. Turn and cook the other side for 2 to 3 minutes, until browned. Serve topped with the cottage cheese, fruit, and applesauce.

NUTRITIONAL INFORMATION PER SERVING:

407 calories · 27g protein · 53g carbohydrates · 8g fiber · 9g fat · 1g saturated fat · 176mg sodium

⭐ VEGGIE–EGG WHITE FRITTATA

This savory frittata (an Italian-style omelet that's browned on both sides) is packed with flavor and nutrition. *1 serving*

4 large egg whites	1 teaspoon finely chopped garlic
½ tablespoon olive oil	4 cherry tomatoes, quartered
¼ cup chopped onion	2 cups fresh spinach, chopped
¼ cup sliced mushrooms	¼ cup water

In a small bowl, beat the egg whites just until white and frothy. In a medium skillet, heat the olive oil over medium heat and sauté the onions, mushrooms, and garlic until they begin to soften. Stir in the tomatoes, spinach, and water, then cover the skillet so the steam from the water cooks the spinach. Once the spinach has wilted and all of the water has been absorbed, pour the egg whites evenly over the vegetables. Cook until top is slightly firm and bottom is browned, turn carefully, and continue to cook until the other side is browned. (You can also finish this frittata under a preheated broiler in about 5 to 6 minutes instead of trying to flip it if you are using an ovenproof skillet. Place the pan on the top shelf and watch the frittata carefully so it doesn't burn.)

NUTRITIONAL INFORMATION PER SERVING:

168 calories · 19g protein · 10g carbohydrates · 4g fiber · 7g fat · 1g saturated fat · 272mg sodium

⭐ CHEESE-Y EGG WHITE OMELET

An egg white omelet makes a delicious breakfast that is packed with goodness. This high-protein version will help your body burn more fat as a fuel source. For lunch or dinner, pair this omelet with a turkey sausage patty, a small salad, or a serving of steamed broccoli or sautéed spinach.

1 serving

½ tablespoon olive oil	2 slices (2.5 ounces) low-sodium turkey
¼ cup chopped onion	breast, chopped

¼ cup chopped mushrooms

4 large egg whites, beaten

¼ cup shredded organic part-skim
mozzarella cheese

In an omelet pan, heat the olive oil over medium heat and sauté the onion until it is translucent. Add the turkey breast and mushrooms and cook for another 3 to 4 minutes. Add the egg whites to the mixture. Raise the heat to moderately high and, using a fork, draw the edges of the mixture in toward the center as it cooks. At the same time, tilt and gently shake the pan so uncooked portions of the egg flow underneath. Cook until the mixture is firm yet creamy. Sprinkle the cheese on top of the mixture, then fold the omelet in half and remove from the pan. Serve on a warmed plate.

NUTRITIONAL INFORMATION PER SERVING:

287 calories · 33g protein · 9g carbohydrates · 1g fiber · 5g fat · 3g saturated fat · 414mg sodium

EGG WHITE–TURKEY SCRAMBLE

This is a favorite breakfast meal among fitness competitors, athletes, and bodybuilders. It is packed full of protein to help you rebuild those muscle fibers and burn fat.

1 serving

4 ounces lean ground turkey

1 fresh basil leaf, chopped, or 1 teaspoon
dried basil

1 fresh sage leaf, chopped, or 1 teaspoon
dried sage

1 pinch sea salt or Himalayan salt

2 teaspoons freshly ground black pepper

¼ cup chopped onion

1 clove garlic, minced

½ tablespoon olive oil

8 cherry tomatoes, quartered

4 large egg whites, beaten

Using clean hands, combine the ground turkey, basil, sage, sea salt, and pepper in a small bowl. In a medium skillet over medium heat, sauté the onion and garlic with half of the olive oil for 1 to 2 minutes. Add the seasoned turkey and continue to cook, until the turkey is cooked through, stirring constantly. Add the cherry tomatoes and cook for 1 minute. Remove the turkey mixture from the skillet with a slotted spoon and discard any excess fat, wiping the skillet with paper towel. Lightly coat the skillet with the remaining olive oil and heat again over medium. Return the turkey mixture to the skillet, add the egg whites, and sauté for 2 minutes, or until the egg whites are completely cooked.

NUTRITIONAL INFORMATION PER SERVING:

334 calories · 37g protein · 8g carbohydrates · 15g fat · 4g saturated fat · 820mg sodium · 0g fiber

CHEF RONNDA'S TURKEY SAUSAGE PATTIES

Chef Ronnda is an internationally trained gourmet chef who has personally cooked and catered for some of Hollywood's A-list. She is well known throughout Hollywood for her healthy and delicious food-delivery program, Chomp Gourmet. Ronnda's Turkey Sausage Patties are among my favorite breakfast sidekicks. Mouthwatering and nutritious, this recipe makes 10 patties, so be sure to limit yourself to just one or two and freeze the rest for your next breakfast or quick snack. *10 patties*

1 pound ground turkey breast, 7% fat
1 egg white
1 tablespoon olive oil
3 fresh basil leaves, chopped
2 fresh sage leaves, chopped

1 clove garlic, minced
4 teaspoons sea salt
5 teaspoons freshly ground black pepper
Cooking spray

In a medium bowl, mix all the ingredients thoroughly. Form the mixture into 2½-inch patties. Brown the patties, in batches if needed, in a heavy skillet coated with cooking spray over moderately high heat, about 3 to 4 minutes per side, or until done. Or place on a heavy baking pan coated with cooking spray and bake at 350° F for 10 minutes.

NUTRITIONAL INFORMATION PER PATTY:

112 calories · 13g protein · 6g fat · 2g saturated fat · 370mg sodium · 0g carbohydrates · 0g fiber

GUILT-FREE BREAKFAST QUESADILLA

The wide variety of cheese in the dairy department can become confusing, so keep in mind that organic cheese and other organic milk products come from cows that have not been injected with hormones and that feed on grass that has not been treated with chemical pesticides or herbicides. One of my favorite cheeses for this recipe is an organic reduced-fat Monterey Jack. Instead of low-fat sour cream for dipping, I have chosen plain Greek yogurt, which very much resembles the taste of sour cream but it is lower in calories and higher in protein, and contains active bacteria cultures. If you feel you need one more tablespoon, go ahead—it's guilt free!

1 serving

4 large egg whites
½ tablespoon olive oil
¼ cup chopped onion
1 small jalapeño pepper, seeded and diced
¼ cup diced red and yellow bell peppers
¼ cup shredded organic reduced-fat
   Monterey Jack cheese

2 (6-inch) whole wheat tortillas
2 teaspoons freshly ground pepper
2 tablespoons bottled salsa
2 tablespoons Greek yogurt

In a small bowl, beat the egg whites until blended and frothy. In a medium skillet, warm the olive oil over medium heat. Sauté the onion and peppers for 1 minute and then add the egg whites and half of the cheese. Continue to cook without stirring until the egg mixture is firm, then turn and cook until the other side is lightly browned. Remove the eggs to a heated plate and set aside. Place one tortilla in the pan and top with the cooked eggs. Sprinkle the remaining cheese and ground pepper over the eggs and top with the second tortilla. Immediately turn, cook for about 15 seconds, and remove from heat. Cut the quesadilla into quarters and serve with the salsa and yogurt on the side for dipping.

NUTRITIONAL INFORMATION PER SERVING:

417 calories · 32g protein · 36g carbohydrates · 17g fiber · 12g fat · 4g saturated fat · 880mg sodium

WHOLE WHEAT BREAKFAST BURRITO

Breakfast burritos are a great option for those mornings when you want to start your day with a little spice. They are also perfect when you need something "on the go." *1 serving*

3 large egg whites
½ tablespoon olive oil
1 low-fat turkey sausage (about 3 oz.)
¼ cup chopped onion

1 (6-inch) whole wheat tortilla
8 cherry tomatoes, halved
Cooking spray
2 tablespoons bottled salsa

In a small bowl, beat the egg whites. In a small skillet, heat ¼ tablespoon of the olive oil over medium heat. Brown the turkey sausage for about 8 minutes, until cooked through. Remove from the pan and slice into pieces. In the same pan, heat the remaining ¼ tablespoon of olive oil and sauté the onion until translucent. Add the egg whites and scramble until cooked. Remove the skillet from the heat, add the turkey sausage and cherry tomatoes, cover, and set aside as you prepare the tortilla. In a large skillet sprayed with cooking spray, warm the tortilla on both sides. Place the tortilla on a flat surface, mound the egg mixture in the center of the tortilla, top with the salsa, and roll into a burrito.

NUTRITIONAL INFORMATION PER SERVING:

367 calories · 28g protein · 35g carbohydrates · 10g fiber · 13g fat · 3g saturated fat · 945mg sodium

EGG BLT PITA POCKET

A healthier twist to an all-time favorite! *1 serving*

1 (6½-inch) whole wheat pita pocket
2 eggs, poached firm (see recipe for
    Fast-and-Easy Poached Eggs)

4 slices tomato
2 romaine lettuce leaves
2 slices turkey bacon, cooked

Cut pita in half and fill each pocket with one poached egg, two slices tomato, one lettuce leaf, and one slice turkey bacon.

NUTRITIONAL INFORMATION PER SERVING:

418 calories · 24g protein · 40g carbohydrates · 10g fiber · 17g fat · 5g saturated fat · 878mg sodium

SMOKED SALMON BAGEL WITH A "SCHMEAR"

Salmon is low in saturated fat yet high in protein and a unique type of health-promoting fat, the omega-3 essential fatty acids. As their name implies, essential fatty acids are necessary for good health but because they cannot be made by the body, they must be obtained from foods. Wild-caught cold-water fish like salmon are higher in omega-3 fatty acids than warm-water fish. In addition to its high concentration of omega-3s, salmon is an excellent source of the B vitamins B_{12} and niacin, and the trace mineral selenium. Use an organic low-fat cream cheese as the "schmear" to create this popular brunch favorite. *1 serving*

1 medium whole wheat bagel
2 tablespoons low-fat cream cheese
3 ounces smoked salmon (4 small slices)
2–3 slices tomato
¼ fresh lemon

Cut the bagel in half and toast. Top each half with the cream cheese, salmon, and tomato. Season with the juice from the lemon.

NUTRITIONAL INFORMATION PER SERVING:

329 calories · 26g protein · 36g carbohydrates · 6g fiber · 10g fat · 4g saturated fat · 891mg sodium

CINNAMON BERRY FRENCH TOAST

French toast can be healthy. Just substitute whole wheat bread for the usual white bread, add some extra egg whites to pump up the protein, and top with mixed berries instead of syrup. If you just can't live without the maple syrup, then use just a couple of tablespoons. The nutritional count of this recipe does not include the syrup, so don't forget to factor in the additional calories. (One tablespoon of pure maple syrup is 52 calories.) I recommend real maple syrup over the sugar-free variety because the artificial sweeteners contain chemicals that may contribute to other long-term side effects. *1 serving*

1 large egg

2 large egg whites

¼ cup low-fat milk

1 teaspoon ground cinnamon

½ tablespoon olive oil

2 slices whole wheat bread

1 cup mixed berries (sliced strawberries, blueberries, blackberries, raspberries)

In a medium bowl, beat the egg and egg whites. Add the milk and cinnamon and continue to beat until completely blended. In a medium skillet or griddle pan, warm the olive oil over medium heat. Dip each piece of whole wheat bread into the egg mixture until the bread is completely covered and absorbs some of the mixture. Panfry each piece of bread on both sides on medium-low heat until golden brown. Serve with a topping of the mixed berries.

NUTRITIONAL INFORMATION PER SERVING:

397 calories · 22g protein · 44g carbohydrates · 8g fiber · 15g fat · 3g saturated fat · 352mg sodium

BLUE CORN PANCAKES WITH FRUIT

This recipe uses Arrowhead Mills Blue Corn Pancakes, but you can use another brand if it is not available at your grocery store. Just make sure you read the ingredients and choose organic whenever possible. Blue corn is less refined than white flour, so this is a healthier, great-tasting alternative to buttermilk pancakes. *3 servings (six 5-inch pancakes)*

1 cup dry blue corn pancake mix	1½ tablespoons oil
¾ cup organic low-fat milk	1 banana, sliced
1 large egg	1 cup blueberries

Following the instructions on the package for mixing the blue corn pancakes, add half of the banana and blueberries to the mixture. Coat a medium skillet or griddle lightly with the olive oil and heat over medium heat. Pour half of the batter for each pancake into the skillet and cook until bubbles form over the surface, turn gently, and brown the other side. Serve with the remaining banana and blueberries.

NUTRITIONAL INFORMATION PER SERVING:

335 calories · 10g protein · 46g carbohydrates · 7g fiber · 10g fat · 2g saturated fat · 270mg sodium

BLUEBERRY AND BANANA BUCKWHEAT PANCAKES

Try buckwheat pancakes without the syrup, especially if you are diabetic, and savor the natural flavors of the bananas and blueberries. Blue corn and yellow corn pancake mixes are also yummy alternatives and healthier than using refined white flour. *2 servings*

⅔ cup buckwheat pancake mix (Arrowhead Mills) to make four 5-inch pancakes	¾ cup water
	½ cup sliced bananas
	½ cup blueberries
1 egg	1 tablespoon pure maple syrup (optional)
2 teaspoons canola oil	

In a bowl, stir the pancake mix, egg, 1 teaspoon of canola oil, and water until all of the lumps disappear. Add half of the bananas and blueberries to the mixture. In a medium heavy skillet or griddle pan, heat the remaining canola oil over medium heat. (Or eliminate the oil if you are using a nonstick pan and heat the pan until a drop of water dances on the surface.) Cook until bubbles form on the surface, turn gently, and brown the other side. To serve, top the pancakes with the remaining bananas and blueberries.

NUTRITIONAL INFORMATION PER SERVING (TWO 5-INCH PANCAKES):

396 calories · 8g protein · 90g carbohydrates · 10g fiber · 2g fat · 2g saturated fat · 580mg sodium

FRUIT PLATTER WITH COTTAGE CHEESE

Pink grapefruit, mixed berries, and mango are all rich in phytonutrients, which reduce the risk for cancer, stroke, flu, tooth decay, heart disease, and other, age-related degenerative diseases, as well as antioxidant protection of body fluids such as blood. *1 serving*

½ pink grapefruit, peeled and cut into sections
1 cup mixed berries (blueberries, raspberries, sliced strawberries)
½ mango, sliced
1 cup low-fat, low-sodium cottage cheese

Arrange fruit on a plate and place cottage cheese in the center.

NUTRITIONAL INFORMATION PER SERVING:

309 calories · 28g protein · 43g carbohydrates · 7g fiber · 2g fat · 30mg sodium · 0g saturated fat

GREEK YOGURT CRUNCH

Here is another great meal you can take on the go. Greek yogurt is very low in sugar and high in protein, so it's a perfect choice for those who are diabetic or for anyone who wants to limit their intake of refined sugars. FAGE Greek yogurt is the brand that I see most often at grocery stores. FAGE is the leading dairy company in Greece (www.fageusa.com). Another company, 3 Greek Gods (www.3greekgods.com), also makes organic Greek yogurt. Use your favorite organic low-fat crunchy cereal as a good alternative to low-fat granola and wheat germ. Remember to look for at least 5 grams of fiber or more per serving. Nature's Path is one of my favorite organic cereal brands, and offers a great healthy selection especially for kids as well (www.naturespath.com). *1 serving*

1 cup fat-free Greek yogurt

¼ cup low-fat granola

½ cup mixed berries (blueberries, raspberries, blackberries)

2 tablespoons toasted wheat germ

Pour the yogurt into a medium bowl or travel container and top with granola, berries, and wheat germ.

NUTRITIONAL INFORMATION PER SERVING:

335 calories · 31g protein · 50g carbohydrates · 8g fiber · 32g fat · 175mg sodium · 0g saturated fat

JEANETTE'S CALIFORNIA SUNSHINE PROTEIN SMOOTHIE

A smoothie is an excellent choice if you must have breakfast on the go. When picking one up at the gym or local smoothie shop, be sure to ask about all of the ingredients that are added so you don't get one filled with sugar and a few hundred extra calories. Some of my favorite meal-replacement shakes and supplements that are packed full of nutrients are available from Isagenix Isalean Shake (www.isagenix.com), Living Fuel Rx SuperGreens (www.livingfuel.com), and Udo Erasmus's Wholesome Fast Food (www.udoerasmus.com). But it only takes a few minutes to make a shake at home. Not only will you know exactly what's going into your shake, but you'll also have one bursting with flavor that you won't find in any powdered mix.

1 serving

About 1 cup ice

1½ cups water

1 ounce vanilla whey protein (The goal is
    to get 25 to 30 grams of protein, so you
    may need more than 1 ounce
    depending on the brand.)

½ banana, sliced

½ cup orange juice

1 cup mixed berries

Put the ice and water in the blender and top with the vanilla whey protein, banana, orange juice, and mixed berries. Blend on high speed for 1 to 3 minutes, or until smooth.

NUTRITIONAL INFORMATION PER SERVING:

327 calories · 32g protein · 51g carbohydrates · 6g fiber · 2g fat · 1mg sodium · 0g saturated fat

NUTTY BANANA PROTEIN SMOOTHIE

This shake will satisfy anyone's cravings for peanut butter. There are many tasty nutty spreads, so try something new instead of peanut butter. Nuts also contain healing phytonutrients, so mix them up. My two favorite spreads are soy nut butter and sunflower seed butter. Soy nuts and sunflower seeds contain the healthy fat that your body cannot produce on its own. Most conventional peanut butters contain genetically modified peanuts, hydrogenated oils, and trans fats, so read labels and choose organic with only peanuts in the ingredients. You can use organic low-fat milk, vanilla soy milk, or plain soy milk to make this smoothie, but keep the sugar content below 15 grams per serving. Remember, you have to keep your processed sugar intake to a minimum so you can burn off that body fat. *1 serving*

About 1 cup ice

1 cup organic low-fat milk

1 tablespoon soy nut butter

2 tablespoons protein powder

1 banana, sliced

Put the ice and milk in the blender and top with the soy nut butter, protein powder, and banana. Blend on high speed for 1 to 2 minutes, or until smooth.

NUTRITIONAL INFORMATION PER SERVING:

394 calories · 33g protein · 50g carbohydrates · 5g fiber · 9g fat · 2g saturated fat · 196mg sodium

CURRIED CHICKEN SANDWICH

This combination of curry, walnuts, and raisins is one of my favorites. I admit that I do have a bit of a sweet tooth, and the raisins definitely satisfy my cravings. *1 serving*

2 tablespoons light mayonnaise

¼ teaspoon curry powder

4 ounces boneless, skinless chicken breast, grilled and chopped

16 walnut halves, chopped

14 raisins or currants

½ cup mixed green baby lettuces

2 slices whole wheat bread

In a medium bowl, mix the mayonnaise and curry until combined. Add the chicken, walnuts, and raisins or currants and stir again until all of the ingredients are blended. Place the lettuce on one slice of bread. Top the lettuce with the chicken salad and the remaining bread slice. Cut in half and serve.

NUTRITIONAL INFORMATION PER SERVING:

475 calories · 35g protein · 42g carbohydrates · 7g fiber · 20g fat · 2g saturated fat · 505mg sodium

CHICKEN TOMATO AVOCADO PITA

I know people are often confused about whether avocados are healthy because they are high in fat. Yes they are healthy, very healthy. Ninety percent of an avocado's calories come from monounsaturated fat that helps you control your appetite and lose weight. The monounsaturated fat in avocados speeds up your basal metabolic rate, which makes you feel full faster and helps reduce overeating. The high fat content in avocados also helps you resist the temptation to binge on foods high in sugar or saturated fats. Avocados are also full of the antioxidants that help protect us against arthritis, cancer, cataracts, heart disease, and even the effects of aging. They provide more than twenty-five essential nutrients, including fiber, potassium, vitamin E, B vitamins, and folic acid. Don't be fooled by fat-free diets—avocados are healthy and they will help you lose weight. *1 serving*

1 (6-inch) whole wheat pita
½ cup mixed green baby lettuces
6 ounces boneless, skinless chicken breast, grilled and sliced
½ small avocado (about 1 ounce), sliced
1 medium tomato, sliced

Slice the pita in half and put half of the ingredients in each pocket.

NUTRITIONAL INFORMATION PER SERVING:

437 calories · 43g protein · 45g carbohydrates · 8g fiber · 10g fat · 2g saturated fat · 787mg sodium

CHICKEN FAJITAS

You can try a different source of protein each time you make fajitas. This recipe calls for chicken, but you can also use a lean cut of steak, seitan, or extra-firm tofu. First start with your favorite and then next time, try something new. If you decide to use a prepared marinade, check the ingredients carefully to make sure you are not getting too much sugar or sodium. (The nutritional information for this recipe includes the homemade marinade.) *4 servings*

MARINADE
¼ cup white wine vinegar
2 tablespoons balsamic vinegar
¼ cup olive oil

1 teaspoon cayenne pepper, or to taste
3 cloves garlic, minced
¼ teaspoon ground cumin

1 tablespoon freshly ground black pepper

2 tablespoons lime juice

1 tablespoon orange juice

1 tablespoon lemon juice

FILLING

16 ounces boneless, skinless chicken
    breast, cut into strips

1 tablespoon olive oil

1 large sweet onion, cut into strips

1 green bell pepper, cut into strips

1 red bell pepper, cut into strips

2 tablespoons chopped cilantro

4 (6-inch) whole wheat tortillas

ACCOMPANIMENTS

4 tablespoons guacamole, or 8 avocado slices

4 ounces fat-free Greek yogurt

8 tablespoons bottled salsa (I recommend Amy's Organic Salsa, medium)

2 limes, sliced into a total of 8 wedges

For the marinade: In a large bowl, mix all of the ingredients until well combined.

For the fajitas: Marinate the chicken strips for at least 30 minutes. In a very large skillet, heat the oil over high heat. Sauté the onion and peppers for about 8 minutes, or until crisp-tender, then remove them from the pan and set aside. Add the chicken and all of the marinade to the skillet and cook, stirring constantly, until the chicken is thoroughly done. Return the vegetables to the skillet with the chicken and add the cilantro. Cook until everything is thoroughly heated, stirring constantly.

Just before serving, wrap the tortillas in foil and heat them in the oven for 10 minutes or in a separate skillet for about 30 seconds on each side or until lightly toasted. Place ¼ of the chicken mixture in each tortilla, roll up, and serve with the guacamole or avocado slices, Greek yogurt, salsa, and lime wedges.

NUTRITIONAL INFORMATION PER SERVING (MARINADE ONLY):

138 calories · 1g protein · 4g carbohydrates · 14g fat · 2g saturated fat · 340mg sodium · 0g fiber

NUTRITIONAL INFORMATION PER SERVING (INCLUDES MARINADE):

443 calories · 35g protein · 27g carbohydrates · 10g fiber · 7g fat · 2g saturated fat · 876mg sodium

FISH TACOS

Once you try fish tacos you'll be a convert to the traditional fast food of California beach towns. This recipe calls for halibut, but you can use another fish such as sole, tilapia, or sea bass if halibut is not available at your grocery store. *4 servings*

3 tablespoons canola oil

Juice of 1 lime

1 clove garlic, minced

1 teaspoon annatto powder

1 small jalapeño pepper, seeded and sliced

16 ounces halibut fillet

4 (6-inch) whole wheat tortillas

1 cup shredded cabbage

1 cup shredded carrots

¼ cup chopped cilantro

½ cup diced red onion

½ cup of your favorite bottled salsa
   (I like Amy's Organic Salsa, medium)

4 ounces fat-free Greek yogurt

1 lime, cut into 4 wedges for juicing

In a small bowl, mix the oil, lime juice, garlic, annatto, and jalapeño to make a marinade. Place the fish in a glass baking dish and pour the marinade over the fish. Cover and refrigerate for 20 minutes.

Preheat an electric or gas grill (or a ribbed cast-iron "grilling" pan on a stove top) to medium to high heat. Remove the halibut from the marinade and grill each side for 4 to 5 minutes, or until the fish is opaque and slightly charred on both sides. Remove from the heat and allow to cool for 5 minutes. Cut the fish into four thick slices.

Heat the tortillas directly on the grill, about 15 seconds per side, or until lightly toasted and warm. Mound the fish, cabbage, carrots, cilantro, onion, salsa, and yogurt, and season with a squeeze of fresh lime juice. Wrap the tortillas to serve.

NUTRITIONAL INFORMATION PER SERVING:

377 calories · 38g protein · 23g carbohydrates · 10g fiber · 15g fat · 1g saturated fat · 712mg sodium

SALMON SALAD SANDWICH

Canned salmon is an easy, convenient way to get all of the healthy benefits of fresh salmon. Always choose the water-packed variety. *1 serving*

2 tablespoons light mayonnaise

6 ounces canned wild salmon, packed
   in water

8 cherry tomatoes, chopped

½ small sweet onion, chopped

1 teaspoon freshly ground black pepper

½ cup mixed green baby lettuce

2 slices whole wheat bread

In a medium bowl, mix the mayonnaise, salmon, tomatoes, onion, and pepper until combined. Place the lettuce on one slice of bread. Top the lettuce with the salmon salad and the remaining bread slice. Cut in half and serve.

NUTRITIONAL INFORMATION PER SERVING:

463 calories · 38g protein · 45g carbohydrates · 7g fiber · 15g fat · 3g saturated fat · 1,283mg sodium

TUNA PITA SANDWICH

Tuna is a cold-water fish that is packed with lean protein and healthy omega-3 fatty acids that your body cannot produce on its own but must get through food. The brain is composed of more than 60 percent fat, and many brain disorders, including Alzheimer's, depression, memory loss, and attention deficit disorders, have been linked to a deficiency in omega-3 fatty acids. Of course you all know the amazing benefits that omega-3 fatty acid fish oils have on decreasing your risk of cardiovascular disease, stroke, blood clots, and certain types of cancer (breast, colon, and prostate). So enjoy that tuna sandwich knowing that you are helping the health of your body. *1 serving*

1 (5.8-ounce) can albacore tuna, packed
   in water

8 cherry tomatoes, chopped

1 small onion, thinly sliced

½ teaspoon freshly ground black pepper

½ tablespoon olive oil

1 (6-inch) whole wheat pocket pita

½ cup mixed green baby lettuce

In a small bowl, mix the tuna, tomatoes, onion, ground pepper, and olive oil until combined. Cut the pita in half and fill each pocket with half of the lettuce and tuna mixture.

NUTRITIONAL INFORMATION PER SERVING:

477 calories · 51g protein · 48g carbohydrates · 8g fiber · 8g fat · 1g saturated fat · 910mg sodium

TUNA SALAD WRAP

A tuna wrap is a great high-protein lunch that you can prepare the night before and throw into a brown bag for your lunch the next day. *1 serving*

1 (5.8-ounce) can albacore tuna,
   packed in water

2 tablespoons light mayonnaise

¼ cup diced red and yellow bell peppers

8 cherry tomatoes, diced

¼ cup chopped celery

¼ cup chopped onion

½ teaspoon freshly ground black pepper

½ cup mixed green baby lettuce

1 (6-inch) whole wheat tortilla

In a small bowl, mix the tuna, mayonnaise, peppers, tomatoes, celery, onion, and pepper until combined. Place the lettuce and the tuna mixture in the center of the whole wheat tortilla and fold bottom half of tortilla over the mixture. Tuck in both ends and continue to roll until wrap is closed. Cut in half and serve or pack in lunch bag.

NUTRITIONAL INFORMATION PER SERVING:

413 calories · 48g protein · 30g carbohydrates · 12g fiber · 11g fat · 1g saturated fat · 1,053mg sodium

TURKEY BLT PITA POCKET

1 serving

1 (6½-inch) whole wheat pita pocket
½ tablespoon light canola mayonnaise
3 slices turkey bacon, cooked and cut into halves
4 slices tomato
2 leaves romaine lettuce

Cut pita in half and spread mayonnaise lightly inside each pita half. Fill each pocket with 3 pieces of cut turkey bacon, 2 slices of tomato, and 1 leaf of lettuce.

NUTRITIONAL INFORMATION PER SERVING:
282 calories • 14g protein • 37g carbohydrates • 7g fiber •
11g fat • 4g saturated fat • 816mg sodium

TURKEY BURGER

Sprouted-grain bread has more nutrients than regular whole wheat or white bread because the grain has fully grown and matured before it is harvested and used to make bread. *1 serving*

4 ounces lean ground turkey
1 sprouted grain burger bun
½ cup mixed green baby lettuce

2 slices tomato
3 teaspoons mustard
1 tablespoon ketchup

Form the lean ground turkey into a round patty. Preheat a nonstick skillet over medium heat. Add the patty and sauté until both sides are golden brown and the middle is cooked through. Remove the patty from the skillet. Warm the burger bun in the skillet or a toaster oven until slightly toasted, then remove it and place the patty on the bun. Garnish with lettuce, tomato, mustard, and ketchup.

NUTRITIONAL INFORMATION PER SERVING:

375 calories · 30g protein · 38g carbohydrates · 7g fiber · 11g fat · 3g saturated fat · 623mg sodium

TURKEY PITA SANDWICH

Quick, easy, and healthy! *1 serving*

1 (6-inch) whole wheat pita pocket
3 teaspoons mustard
4 slices free-range turkey breast
4 slices tomato
½ cup mixed green baby lettuces

Cut the pita in half and spread the mustard inside each pocket. Place half of the turkey, tomato, and lettuce into each pita half.

NUTRITIONAL INFORMATION PER SERVING:

308 calories · 22g protein · 50g carbohydrates · 7g fiber · 4g fat · 1g saturated fat · 553mg sodium

Variation

For an easy alternative that will add a boost of healthy fat, protein, and fiber, substitute 4 tablespoons of hummus for the mustard.

NUTRITIONAL INFORMATION PER SERVING:

391 calories · 26g protein · 56g carbohydrates · 11g fiber · 9g fat · 1g saturated fat · 597mg sodium

SOFT TURKEY TACO

Mexican food is always a favorite, but the way it's often served in local restaurants is not always the best choice when it comes to healthy eating. With a few substitutions, this taco is now low in saturated fat, high in protein and fiber, and ready for you to enjoy. By avoiding the frying that is often associated with tacos, you also eliminate the saturated fat that is traditionally used.

This recipe yields one taco but it is very simple to just multiply the ingredients according to the number of servings you wish to make. *1 serving*

4 ounces lean ground turkey
¼ cup chopped onion
1 clove garlic, minced
¼ cup diced red and yellow bell peppers
4 tablespoons of your favorite salsa
2 teaspoons low-sodium taco seasoning
1 (6-inch) whole wheat tortilla

¼ cup shredded reduced-fat Monterey
   Jack cheese
2 tablespoons nonfat Greek yogurt
8 cherry tomatoes, diced, or
   ½ tomato, diced
½ cup mixed green baby lettuce

In a prewarmed medium skillet, combine the turkey, onion, garlic, peppers, 2 tablespoons of salsa, and the taco seasoning. Cook on medium heat until the turkey is browned, then remove from heat and drain off any excess fat.

In a clean, heavy skillet over medium-high heat, warm the tortilla about 15 seconds on each side, or until it is lightly toasted. Remove the tortilla from the skillet and mound the turkey mixture, cheese, the remaining salsa, yogurt, diced tomatoes, and lettuce in the middle and fold from top and bottom to form the taco.

NUTRITIONAL INFORMATION PER SERVING:

429 calories · 37g protein · 36g carbohydrates · 11g fiber · 15g fat · 3g saturated fat · 1,259mg sodium

BLACK BEAN AND CORN SALAD

This salad is one of my favorite side dishes to pair with fish. Black beans and corn both have lots of fiber, leaving you feeling full and satisfied. The fiber will also slow down the absorption of sugar into your bloodstream, so you will continue to burn fat. Black beans are an especially good choice for diabetics. *4 servings*

1 (14-ounce) can black beans, rinsed and drained

2 cups canned corn kernels, drained

1 medium red bell pepper, seeded and chopped

1 medium tomato, chopped

1 small red onion, chopped

1½ teaspoons ground cumin

1 teaspoon bottled hot sauce

Juice of 1 lime

1 tablespoon olive oil

1 tablespoon ground coriander

1 teaspoon freshly ground black pepper

In a large bowl, toss all of the ingredients until well combined. Let stand for 15 minutes to allow flavors to blend. Serve as a side dish or as a snack.

NUTRITIONAL INFORMATION PER SERVING:

226 calories · 11g protein · 35g carbohydrates · 9g fiber · 2g fat · 313mg sodium · 0 saturated fat

CRANBERRY WALNUT SALAD

This flavorful salad goes particularly well as a side dish with chicken, turkey, or a white fish or on its own as a snack. *1 serving*

1 cup mixed greens

8 walnut halves, chopped

2 tablespoons dried cranberries

2 tablespoons low-fat feta cheese

2 tablespoons low-fat balsamic dressing (Trader Joe's fat-free or Whole Foods low-fat balsamic dressing)

In a small sealable container, mix all of the ingredients and shake vigorously until the contents are combined. Serve with a main dish or as a snack.

NUTRITIONAL INFORMATION PER SERVING:

190 calories · 17g carbohydrates · 3g fiber · 5g protein · 12g fat · 3g saturated fat · 706mg sodium

ASIAN CHICKEN–CABBAGE SALAD

Cabbage is part of the same family as broccoli and, just like broccoli, is packed with cancer-fighting phytonutrients and vitamins. This salad can be a main dish or a healthy, tasty snack because it is well balanced with protein, carbohydrates, and fat. You can use either cooked turkey or chicken for this recipe—perfect for using holiday dinner leftovers. *4 servings*

1 tablespoon sesame seeds, toasted
1½ tablespoons slivered almonds
½ large cabbage, thinly sliced
2 finely chopped green onions
12 ounces boneless, skinless chicken
    breasts, cooked and roughly chopped

⅓ cup unsweetened pineapple juice
¼ cup rice wine vinegar
1 tablespoon low-sodium soy sauce
2 teaspoons sugar
1 tablespoon toasted sesame oil
¼ teaspoon freshly ground black pepper

In a large bowl, mix the sesame seeds, almonds, cabbage, onions, and chicken until combined.

In a separate bowl, mix the pineapple juice, rice wine vinegar, soy sauce, sugar, sesame oil, and pepper until combined. Pour over the salad mixture and toss lightly. Chill overnight to let the flavors blend.

NUTRITIONAL INFORMATION PER SERVING:

208 calories · 24g protein · 14g carbohydrates · 8g fiber · 7g fat · 1g saturated fat · 237mg sodium

CHINESE CHICKEN SALAD

Everyone loves a great Chinese chicken salad because it is light and satisfying, with a wonderful combination of sweet and sour tastes. *4 servings*

¼ cup rice wine vinegar

4 teaspoons sugar

3 tablespoons low-sodium soy sauce

2 tablespoons olive oil

½ tablespoon sesame oil

12 cups mixed salad greens, washed and drained

¼ cup chopped cilantro or parsley

1 pound boneless, skinless chicken breast, cooked and shredded

1 tablespoon sesame seeds

2 small mandarin oranges, peeled and separated

In a large bowl, combine the vinegar, sugar, soy sauce, olive oil, and sesame oil, stirring until the sugar dissolves. Add the salad greens and cilantro to the bowl and toss until evenly coated with the dressing. Add the chicken and toss again. Divide onto four plates. Garnish with the sesame seeds and mandarin oranges.

NUTRITIONAL INFORMATION PER SERVING:

260 calories · 28g protein · 12g carbohydrates · 3g fiber · 10g fat · 2g saturated fat · 534mg sodium

QUICK-AND-EASY CHICKEN CAESAR SALAD

Choose a healthy Caesar dressing to make this salad complete. I recommend Annie's Naturals Caesar dressing and Newman's Own organic creamy Caesar dressing, but remember to compare the brands and read the lists of ingredients. For convenience, you can grill the chicken on a countertop electric grill. (See Grilled Chicken Breasts recipe.) *1 serving*

4 ounces boneless, skinless chicken breast, grilled and chopped

5 cups chopped romaine lettuce (about ½ a head)

2 tablespoons bottled Caesar dressing

2 teaspoons freshly ground black pepper

1 tablespoon grated Parmesan cheese

Juice of ¼ fresh lemon

In a sealable container, mix all of the ingredients except the lemon juice and shake vigorously for 20 to 30 seconds, until combined. Turn out onto a plate and sprinkle with the lemon juice.

NUTRITIONAL INFORMATION PER SERVING:

302 calories · 33g protein · 10g carbohydrates · 5g fiber · 14g fat · 2g saturated fat · 335mg sodium

CHICKEN CRANBERRY NUT SALAD

The cranberries will add an appealing sweet flavor to this refreshing, easy-to-prepare salad. You might like to substitute other fruit such as pear, grapes, raisins, mandarin orange, or apple.

1 serving

4 ounces boneless, skinless chicken breast, grilled and chopped

3–4 cups mixed green baby lettuce

¼ cup reduced-fat feta cheese, crumbled

¼ cup dried cranberries

16 walnut halves

¼ medium red onion, diced

3 tablespoons low-fat or fat-free balsamic dressing

In a large bowl, combine all the ingredients until well coated with the dressing.

NUTRITIONAL INFORMATION PER SERVING:

485 calories · 36g protein · 36g carbohydrates · 6g fiber · 22g fat · 4g saturated fat · 557mg sodium

GREEK CHICKEN SALAD

Enjoy this light and delicious salad with half a pita or a small cup of lentil soup for additional fiber. If you wish, use salmon instead of chicken, but be sure to change the nutritional counts if you substitute (see chart, pp. 246–254). *2 servings*

8 ounces boneless, skinless chicken
   breast, cooked and chopped
1 cup sliced cucumber
4 tablespoons sliced pitted black olives
¼ cup reduced-fat feta cheese, crumbled

1 medium tomato, chopped
¼ small red onion, chopped
4 tablespoons Greek or Italian low-fat
   salad dressing
6 cups mixed green baby lettuce

In a large bowl, lightly mix the chicken, cucumber, olives, feta, tomato, and onion until combined. Add the salad dressing and coat well. Cover and refrigerate for at least 1 hour to allow the flavors to blend. Divide the greens onto two plates, mound the chicken mixture on each, and serve.

NUTRITIONAL INFORMATION PER SERVING:

319 calories · 33g protein · 12g carbohydrates · 4g fiber · 14g fat · 2g saturated fat · 483mg sodium

CURRIED CHICKEN SALAD

One of my favorite fat-free balsamic dressings is made by Trader Joe's, but since balsamic dressing is so popular you will find a good selection in your grocery store. Remember to compare the ingredients and calorie total. *1 serving*

2 tablespoons light mayonnaise
¼ teaspoon curry powder
4 ounces boneless, skinless chicken
   breast, grilled and chopped
16 walnut halves, chopped

14 raisins or currants
3 cups mixed green baby lettuce
1 medium tomato, chopped
2 tablespoons fat-free balsamic salad
   dressing

In a medium bowl, mix the mayonnaise and curry powder until combined. Add the chicken, walnuts, and raisins or currants and stir until evenly coated. Place the lettuce on a plate and top with the chicken salad and chopped tomato. Sprinkle with the balsamic dressing.

NUTRITIONAL INFORMATION PER SERVING:

399 calories · 31g protein · 71g carbohydrates · 9g fiber · 19g fat · 3g saturated fat · 656mg sodium

MIXED GREENS SALAD

A traditional mixed greens salad is a quick and easy way to guarantee that you load up on vitamins, minerals, fiber, and phytonutrients. It is the perfect complement to any meal, including eggs and breakfast dishes. *1 serving*

- 1 cup mixed greens
- 1 medium tomato, diced
- 4 cucumber slices, cut in halves
- 2 teaspoons chopped red onion
- 2 tablespoons balsamic vinegar
- 1 teaspoon olive oil
- ¼ teaspoon freshly ground black pepper
- 1 tablespoon grated Parmesan cheese

Mix the mixed greens, tomato, cucumber, onion, vinegar, oil, and pepper. In a small sealable container, shake until the contents are blended. Sprinkle with the Parmesan cheese and serve.

NUTRITIONAL INFORMATION PER SERVING:

123 calories · 4g protein · 13g carbohydrates · 3g fiber · 6g fat · 1g saturated fat · 77mg sodium

PEAR–PINE NUT SALAD

Pine nuts are a good source of iron and also contain heart-healthy phytonutrients and mono-unsaturated fat. You can mix up different types of nuts and seeds in your salads because they all have similar benefits. Experiment with walnuts, almonds, pumpkin seeds, ground flaxseed, sunflower seeds, or peanuts, but always try to use the organic, unsalted varieties.

1 serving

1 cup packed fresh baby spinach,
   washed and stemmed
2 tablespoon pine nuts
½ tablespoon olive oil

¼ small red onion, thinly sliced
½ pear, peeled and thinly sliced
¼ teaspoon freshly ground black pepper
Juice of 1 lemon

In a sealable container, mix all of the ingredients. Shake vigorously until the contents are blended. Serve as a side dish or as a snack.

NUTRITIONAL INFORMATION PER SERVING:

207 calories • 5g protein • 19g carbohydrates • 5g fiber • 7g fat • 1g saturated fat • 25mg sodium

TOMATO CUCUMBER SALAD

I love the flavors that come from mixing tomatoes, feta cheese, cucumbers, and lemon. This makes an ideal side salad for fish or as a snack on its own. *1 serving*

1 medium tomato, diced
2 teaspoons chopped onion
1 cup diced cucumber
½ tablespoon olive oil

Juice of 1 lemon
2 tablespoons low-fat feta cheese
¼ teaspoon freshly ground black pepper
½ tablespoon finely chopped fresh basil

In a small sealable container, mix all of the ingredients. Shake well until everything is mixed together.

NUTRITIONAL INFORMATION PER SERVING:

141 calories · 5g protein · 10g carbohydrates · 3g fiber · 9g fat · 1g saturated fat · 246mg sodium

TOMATO AND RED ONION SALAD

The tomato, which is actually a fruit, is celebrated around the world and is used in several recipes here. Lycopene, the most talked about and researched phytonutrient found in the tomato, has been shown to protect humans from several different types of cancer, including colorectal, prostate, breast, endometrial, lung, and pancreatic. *4 servings*

8 Roma tomatoes, diced	¼ teaspoon salt
½ red onion, diced	¼ teaspoon freshly ground black pepper
1 tablespoon olive oil	2 teaspoons minced fresh oregano
8 tablespoons balsamic vinegar	1 teaspoon Dijon mustard (optional)

Place the tomatoes and onion in a large bowl and drizzle with the olive oil and balsamic vinegar. Season with salt, pepper, and oregano and toss until everything is well combined. Cover the bowl with plastic wrap and refrigerate until ready to serve. If you'd like, you can add a teaspoon of Dijon mustard, which is only 5 additional calories and a great way to spice up the dish.

NUTRITIONAL INFORMATION PER SERVING:

58 calories · 1g protein · 10g carbohydrates · 2g fiber · 4g fat · 1g saturated fat · 160mg sodium

ALBACORE TUNA CHOPPED SALAD

A light and refreshing salad packed full of phytonutrients, healthy fat, and protein. This meal will definitely set you two steps ahead in your weight-loss journey. *1 serving*

1 tablespoon freshly squeezed lemon juice
½ teaspoon sugar
1 clove garlic, minced
¼ teaspoon freshly ground black pepper
1 tablespoon olive oil
1 (3-ounce) can albacore tuna, packed
  in water
1 tablespoon grated Parmesan cheese

3 cups chopped romaine lettuce
½ cucumber, peeled and diced
1 medium tomato, diced
¼ cup chopped onion
¼ cup diced red and yellow bell peppers
1 tablespoon chopped parsley
5 pitted black olives, quartered
¼ cup canned chickpeas

In a large bowl, whisk together the lemon juice, sugar, garlic, and pepper. Add the oil in a stream, whisking until combined to create a dressing. Add all other ingredients to the dressing and toss until well coated.

NUTRITIONAL INFORMATION PER SERVING:

415 calories · 30g protein · 36g carbohydrates · 8g fiber · 20g fat · 2g saturated fat · 740mg sodium

ROASTED ACORN SQUASH

Acorn squash, an orange fleshy vegetable like butternut squash and sweet potato, is loaded with cancer-preventing phytonutrients. Vitamin A is the top nutrient in such vegetables, and research has shown that it will also help protect you against emphysema. If you or a loved one smokes, or if you are exposed to secondhand smoke, then make sure you eat orange fleshy vegetables.

4 servings

2 medium acorn squash

2 tablespoons organic unsalted butter

1 teaspoon freshly grated nutmeg

½ teaspoon salt

¼ teaspoon freshly ground black pepper

Preheat the oven to 375° F. Using a large chef's knife, cut the acorn squash in half lengthwise. Scoop out the seeds and stringy middle with a spoon. Spread the butter over the flesh and sprinkle with the nutmeg.

Place the squash halves on a baking sheet flesh side up and roast for 50 minutes, or until the flesh is just tender. Let cool for 20 minutes, then spoon out the flesh and discard the skin. Mash and stir the squash, then season it with salt and pepper. Serve as a side dish or a snack.

NUTRITIONAL INFORMATION PER SERVING:

149 calories · 2g protein · 22g carbohydrates · 6g fiber · 6g fat · 4g saturated fat · 352mg sodium

ROASTED ASPARAGUS

Asparagus is an excellent source of folate, which is essential for any woman who is considering getting pregnant. Folate is necessary for cellular division and DNA synthesis, and folate deficiencies during pregnancy have been linked to several birth defects. A deficiency of folate, which is also found in green leafy vegetables, is the most common vitamin deficiency in the world.

4 servings

2 bunches medium asparagus
   (approximately 28 spears)

2 tablespoons olive oil

½ teaspoon sea salt

Freshly ground black pepper, to taste

2 tablespoons grated or shaved Parmesan

Preheat the oven to 450° F. Trim the woody ends from the asparagus, usually about 1½ inches from the base. Spread the spears on a baking sheet in a single layer, drizzle with the olive oil, and sprinkle with the sea salt and pepper. Roll the asparagus spears on the baking sheet until they're evenly coated with oil. Roast for 8 to 10 minutes, until lightly browned and tender, giving the pan a good shake about halfway through to turn the asparagus. Arrange on a serving platter and top with the Parmesan. Serve warm or at room temperature.

NUTRITIONAL INFORMATION PER SERVING:

97 calories · 4g protein · 5g carbohydrates · 2g fiber · 2g fat · 1g saturated fat · 351mg sodium

BROCCOLI PARMESAN

Adding Parmesan to broccoli is a healthy way to get a cheesy flavor without all the additional calories. *4 servings*

6 cups roughly chopped fresh broccoli
1 tablespoon olive oil
½ teaspoon sea salt or Himalayan salt
2 teaspoons freshly ground black pepper

8 tablespoons freshly grated Parmesan cheese
Juice of 1 lemon

Preheat the oven to 400° F. In a large bowl, toss the broccoli with the oil, sea salt, and pepper until coated evenly. Arrange the broccoli in a single layer on a nonstick cookie sheet and bake for 10 minutes. Remove the broccoli from the oven and sprinkle the cheese evenly over the top. Bake about 10 more minutes, until the cheese melts and forms a crisp shell over the broccoli. Using a spatula, remove the broccoli to a platter and drizzle with the fresh lemon juice. Serve as a side dish or a snack.

NUTRITIONAL INFORMATION PER SERVING:

116 calories · 8g protein · 9g carbohydrates · 4g fiber · 7g fat · 3g saturated fat · 289mg sodium

ROASTED BRUSSELS SPROUTS

Brussels sprouts are part of the same family as broccoli and cabbage known as *Brassica*. Roasting the vegetables and seasoning with the lemon pepper helps cut the strong flavor of the sprouts. If you've had an aversion to Brussels sprouts in the past, this version should make you a convert.

4 servings

4 cups Brussels sprouts (large sprouts should be cut in half to reduce cooking time)
1 tablespoon olive oil
½ teaspoon salt
1 teaspoon lemon pepper
1 lemon

Preheat the oven to 425° F. In a large bowl, toss the spouts with the oil to coat evenly. Transfer to a baking sheet and season with the salt and lemon pepper. Roast for 20 minutes, remove from oven and turn with a spatula or slotted spoon, and return to oven for 20 more minutes, or until the sprouts are fork-tender. Squeeze lemon juice over the sprouts and serve.

NUTRITIONAL INFORMATION PER SERVING:
86 calories · 4g protein · 11g carbohydrates · 4g fiber · 3g fat · 1g saturated fat · 288mg sodium

BAKED BUTTERNUT SQUASH

Another amazing vegetable loaded with nutrients and absolutely delicious! It is a perfect side for any of your chicken or turkey dishes. *4 servings*

1 medium butternut squash
2 tablespoons organic unsalted butter
½ teaspoon sea salt or Himalayan salt
1 teaspoon freshly ground black pepper
1 teaspoon dried rosemary
1 teaspoon dried thyme

Preheat the oven to 375° F. Using a large chef's knife, cut the squash in half lengthwise and scoop out the seeds with a spoon. Set the halves flesh side down on a cutting board and cut them across their centers.

Place the quartered squash on a baking sheet flesh side up and spread the butter over each piece and sprinkle with the salt, pepper, rosemary, and thyme. Cover with foil and bake for 50 to 60 minutes, or until the squash is very tender.

Let cool for 20 minutes, then spoon out the flesh and discard the skin. Mash and stir the squash, then season with salt and pepper to taste.

NUTRITIONAL INFORMATION PER SERVING:

149 calories · 2g protein · 22g carbohydrates · 2g fiber · 6g fat · 4g saturated fat · 345mg sodium

HONEY-GLAZED CARROTS

These are an all-time favorite for many people. This recipe has less sugar and fewer calories than what you'd find in a restaurant—and it's so easy to prepare. *4 servings*

4 cups baby carrots
3 teaspoons packed light brown sugar
1 tablespoon honey
1 tablespoon organic unsalted butter
½ teaspoon salt

Steam the carrots until firm-tender. Drain the carrots. In a medium saucepan, combine the carrots with the remaining ingredients and cook over medium heat, uncovered, about 3 to 5 minutes, stirring frequently, until the sugar, honey, and butter form a glaze over the carrots.

NUTRITIONAL INFORMATION PER SERVING:

104 calories · 1g protein · 19g carbohydrates · 2g fiber · 3g fat · 2g saturated fat · 316mg sodium

LEMON GREEN BEANS

Green beans have lots of vitamin A, C, K, iron, and folate, like many other green vegetables. This zesty recipe makes for a tasty side dish or snack. *4 servings*

12 ounces green beans, ends trimmed
1 tablespoon organic unsalted butter
1 tablespoon minced shallots
2 ounces pine nuts, approximately 20

1 teaspoon freshly squeezed lemon juice
½ teaspoon salt
½ teaspoon freshly ground black pepper

Steam the green beans until firm-tender. Drain the green beans and pat them dry. In a medium skillet, heat the butter over medium heat until melted. Add the shallots and cook for 1 minute, stirring constantly to keep them from burning. Add the pine nuts and cook, stirring, for an additional minute. Add the green beans and toss for about 1 minute, until ingredients are combined. Add the lemon juice, salt, and pepper and toss again. Remove from heat and serve.

NUTRITIONAL INFORMATION PER SERVING:

133 calories · 5g protein · 9g carbohydrates · 4g fiber · 10g fat · 3g saturated fat · 318mg sodium

GRILLED MIXED VEGETABLES

Grilled mixed vegetables are an ideal side to prepare when you are already at the grill doing meat, poultry, or fish. Not only do grilled vegetables taste great, but you'll also save cleanup time in the kitchen. *4 servings*

2 tablespoons olive oil
¼ cup balsamic vinegar
1 teaspoon dried thyme

1 teaspoon dried oregano
1 teaspoon dried basil
1 teaspoon freshly ground black pepper

1 large onion, sliced into ¼-inch-thick rings

1 large yellow bell pepper, sliced into medium wedges

2 medium zucchini, ends trimmed, sliced lengthwise into ¼-inch-thick strips

1 large red bell pepper, sliced into medium wedges

8 baby portobello mushrooms, cleaned and stems removed

2 medium yellow summer squash, sliced

In a small bowl, mix the oil, vinegar, thyme, oregano, basil, and ground pepper until combined. Brush all sides of the vegetables with the mixture. Grill for 15 minutes on medium heat, or until vegetables are tender.

NUTRITIONAL INFORMATION PER SERVING:

153 calories · 4g protein · 18g carbohydrates · 5g fiber · 7g fat · 1g saturated fat · 23mg sodium

GARLIC RAPINI POTATOES

Rapini is also known as broccoli rabe, broccoletti di rape, broccoletto, broccoli di foglia, cime de rape, and rape. The Chinese grow a similar but milder green, known as choy sum, Chinese broccoli, or Chinese flowering cabbage. Rapini resembles its cousin, broccoli, but has tiny bunches of broccoli-like blossoms on long stems amid lots of large spiky leaves. Rapini is a favorite in Italian cooking, and the combination of rapini and potatoes is a very satisfying and yummy side dish packed with fiber, vitamins A, C, and K, iron, and folate. This dish happens to be one of my mom's favorites. *4 servings*

2 tablespoons olive oil

2 cloves garlic, minced

1 bunch rapini (about 1 pound), 3–4 inches trimmed from the stems

2 medium potatoes, peeled, boiled to firm-tender, and chopped into quarters

In a very large skillet or wok, heat the oil. Add the garlic and cook until it begins to sizzle. Add the rapini in small bunches, as much as you can fit in the skillet or wok at a time, and mix so it becomes coated with oil as it cooks. Add the potatoes and continue cooking and mixing the vegetables until the potatoes begin to brown. Serve warm as a side dish or snack.

NUTRITIONAL INFORMATION PER SERVING:

180 calories · 6g protein · 23g carbohydrates · 5g fiber · 17g fat · 1g saturated fat · 71mg sodium

GARLIC SPINACH

Calorie for calorie, spinach provides more nutrients than any other food. Spinach is packed full of iron, vitamins A, C, and K, folate, magnesium, protein, omega-3 fatty acids, and phytonutrients that fight osteoporosis, heart disease, colon cancer, arthritis, and other diseases at the same time. It is also a versatile vegetable that can be prepared in countless ways on its own or combined with other foods. To read more about spinach or any other of the world's healthiest foods, check out the George Mateljan Foundation World's Healthiest Foods Web site at www.whfoods.org.

4 servings

2 tablespoons olive oil
2 cloves garlic, finely chopped
1 bag or 1 bunch of fresh spinach
   (10 ounces), washed, stemmed,
   and patted dry

½ teaspoon sea salt or Himalayan salt
1 teaspoon freshly ground black pepper
Juice of 1 lemon

In a large skillet, heat the oil over medium-high heat. Stir in the garlic and cook for 15 seconds. Add the spinach, salt, and pepper and toss until well combined. Sauté for about 2 minutes, or until all of the spinach is wilted. Remove from heat, splash with lemon juice, and serve.

NUTRITIONAL INFORMATION PER SERVING:

76 calories · 3g protein · 3g carbohydrates · 2g fiber · 7g fat · 1g saturated fat · 538mg sodium

CURRIED SWEET POTATO

Curry powder, which is actually a mix of several different spices, adds a lively and unusual flavor to the sweet potato without being overpowering. This is a healthy alternative to the traditional holiday fare of candied yams, and you can enjoy it all year long. *4 servings*

2 large sweet potatoes

3 tablespoons honey

3 tablespoons freshly squeezed lemon juice

1½ tablespoons olive oil

1 teaspoon curry powder

1 teaspoon fresh lemon zest

Preheat the oven to 400° F. Peel the potatoes and cut them into ¼-inch-thick slices. In a large bowl, mix the honey, lemon juice, olive oil, curry powder, and lemon zest until combined. Lightly coat a nonstick casserole dish or baking pan with olive oil using a paper towel.

Dip the potato slices into the honey mixture and place them in one or two layers in the prepared dish. Drizzle any remaining honey mixture over the potatoes, cover the dish tightly with foil, and bake for 40 minutes. Remove the foil and continue baking for 20 more minutes, turning the potatoes over after 10 minutes for even browning.

NUTRITIONAL INFORMATION PER SERVING:

177 calories • 2g protein • 33g carbohydrates • 3g fiber • 5g fat • 1g saturated fat • 0mg sodium

HONEY-MUSTARD LAMB CHOPS

This is a simple recipe and a nice change from the regular chicken or fish meal. Prepare this the next time you have guests over and impress them with your unexpected culinary skills. They'll be even more surprised when they find out it's healthy. Of course, that does not mean you can have extra—remember portion control and stick to one serving. *6 servings*

2 tablespoons honey

2 tablespoons freshly squeezed lemon juice

2 tablespoons freshly squeezed orange juice

2 tablespoons minced fresh rosemary

½ teaspoon Dijon mustard

1 teaspoon minced garlic

1 teaspoon onion powder

½ teaspoon dry mustard

6 (5-ounce) lamb chops, trimmed of fat

6 mint sprigs

Preheat the broiler or grill. In a small bowl, mix the honey, lemon juice, orange juice, rosemary, mustard, garlic, onion powder, and dry mustard to create a basting sauce. Brush each side of the lamb chops with the sauce and place on broiler pan or grill. Broil one side 5 to 6 inches from heat source for 6 to 7 minutes, or until brown. Turn chops and brush with remaining sauce and broil for 6 to 7 more minutes, or until brown. (If grilling, baste and turn frequently for 15 to 20 minutes, or until cooked through.) Garnish with mint and serve.

NUTRITIONAL INFORMATION PER SERVING:

314 calories · 38g protein · 7g carbohydrates · 14g fat · 5g saturated fat · 104mg sodium · 0g fiber

APPLE PORK TENDERLOIN

Choose your meat wisely. Always try for organic and make sure there are no added hormones. You can also prepare this recipe with boneless, skinless chicken or turkey. *4 servings*

4 (4-ounce) ½-inch-thick pieces pork tenderloin

1½ tablespoons curry powder

1 tablespoon extra-virgin olive oil

1 medium onion, chopped

2 cups apple cider

1 apple, peeled, seeded, and chopped into chunks

1 tablespoon cornstarch

Season the tenderloins with curry powder on both sides and let stand in the refrigerator for 15 minutes.

In a large skillet, heat the olive oil over medium high heat. Add the tenderloins and cook, 10 to 12 minutes, until browned on both sides, turning once. Remove the meat from the skillet and set aside.

Saute the onions in the skillet until soft and golden. Add 1½ cups of the apple cider, reduce heat to low, and simmer until the liquid reduces to half. Add the chopped apple, sprinkle the cornstarch over the apple, and pour on the remaining ½ cup apple cider. Stir and simmer while the sauce thickens, about 2 minutes. Return the tenderloins to the skillet and simmer for 5 to 10 more minutes, covered. To serve, arrange the tenderloins on a plate, top with the sauce, and serve immediately.

NUTRITIONAL INFORMATION PER SERVING:

309 calories · 32g protein · 24g carbohydrates · 1g fiber · 9g fat · 2g saturated fat · 65mg sodium

BROILED SIRLOIN STEAK

When you are choosing red meat from your grocery store, look for organic beef. Healthy beef can only come from healthy cows. Remember, four ounces of steak is one serving. That's about the size of a deck of cards. Most steaks you get at restaurants are approximately 2 to 4 servings, which contributes to the bad rap that red meat gets simply because our serving sizes are too big and out of control. *1 serving*

3 tablespoons red wine vinegar
1 clove garlic, minced
1 tablespoon Worcestershire sauce
½ tablespoon olive oil

1 (4-ounce) top sirloin steak
1 small onion, sliced
¼ teaspoon dried parsley

In a small bowl, mix the red wine vinegar, garlic, Worcestershire sauce, and olive oil to make a marinade. Place the steak in a sealable plastic bag, pour in the marinade, seal, and refrigerate for at least 30 minutes or as long as overnight.

Preheat the broiler. Cover a grill pan with foil to catch the drippings and then place the grill rack on top of the pan. If you don't have a grill pan, you can use any oven-safe pan. Place the marinated steak topped with the onions on the pan and broil for 10 to 15 minutes, or until the meat reaches your desired level of doneness. Turn the meat after the first 5 minutes. A thick steak is going to require a longer cooking time. Remove steak to a warm plate, garnish with the parsley, and serve.

NUTRITIONAL INFORMATION PER SERVING:

297 calories · 35g protein · 5g carbohydrates · 13g fat · 4g saturated fat · 268mg sodium · 0g fiber

⭐ GRILLED CHICKEN BREASTS

Chicken breasts are an excellent source of protein and can be used in many healthy lunch or dinner dishes. Here's a fast and easy way to prepare them using a countertop grill, to ensure that they'll be moist and juicy. *4 servings*

4 (6-ounce) boneless, skinless chicken
   breasts
¼ cup olive oil
Juice of 1 lemon
1 teaspoon salt

1 teaspoon freshly ground black pepper
Additional seasonings such as garlic,
   rosemary, cilantro, oregano, or basil,
   to taste

Rinse the chicken thoroughly with cool water. Pound each breast with a meat tenderizer to a uniform ½-inch thickness and set aside. In a large bowl, mix the olive oil, lemon juice, salt, pepper, and other seasonings until combined. Immerse the chicken in the marinade, fully coating each piece, remove from marinade, and put chicken in a medium sealable plastic bag, then push air out and seal. Marinate for at least 1 hour in the refrigerator.

Heat the countertop grill until it reaches medium heat. Remove the chicken from the sealable bags and cook, turning after 3 to 4 minutes, for 6 to 8 minutes, or until golden brown.

NUTRITIONAL INFORMATION PER SERVING:

314 calories · 35g protein · 1g carbohydrates · 17g fat · 2g saturated fat · 575mg sodium · 0g fiber

ASIAN CHICKEN STIR-FRY

This is an easy meal to fix when you just don't have a lot of time. When you buy Asian sauces and marinades such as teriyaki, read and compare the ingredients and watch especially for sodium and sugar, which should be as low as possible. Whole Foods, Annie's Naturals (www.anniesnaturals.com), Steel's Gourmet Foods (www.steelsgourmet.com), and other markets have a selection of organic sauces and condiments, including organic teriyaki sauces. Whichever brand you choose, only use up to 100 calories per serving of sauce. *1 serving*

MARINADE

1½ tablespoons grated fresh ginger

1 teaspoon sesame oil

1 teaspoon garlic powder

2 tablespoons Worcestershire sauce

STIR-FRY

2 tablespoons dark sesame oil

1 clove garlic, finely chopped

4 ounces boneless, skinless chicken
breast, cut into strips

2 cups frozen stir-fry vegetables

2 tablespoons homemade marinade or
bottled Asian marinade or teriyaki
sauce

For the marinade: In a small bowl, combine all of the marinade ingredients and mix thoroughly with a metal spoon.

For the stir-fry: In a wok or deep-sided skillet, heat 1 tablespoon of the oil over medium heat. Add the garlic and cook until golden, stirring constantly. Add the chicken and cook for about 4 minutes on each side, or until golden brown. Remove the chicken from the pan and set aside.

In the wok or skillet, heat the remaining tablespoon of oil over medium heat. Add the vegetables and the marinade/teriyaki sauce and stir-fry until the vegetables begin to soften. Stir in the cooked chicken and continue to cook for 2 to 3 minutes. Serve immediately.

NUTRITIONAL INFORMATION PER SERVING:

360 calories · 28g protein · 22g carbohydrates · 4g fiber · 16g fat · 2g saturated fat · 755mg sodium

BAKED LEMON-HERB CHICKEN

The light breading and the lemon give this chicken dish a lot of flavor and zest, but most of the saturated fat has been eliminated by removing the skin and baking the chicken instead of deep frying. *4 servings*

½ cup whole wheat bread crumbs

2 tablespoons grated Parmesan cheese

2 tablespoons sesame seeds

1 teaspoon dried oregano

1 teaspoon dried tarragon

1 teaspoon dried thyme

Grated rind and juice of 1 lemon

¼ teaspoon sea salt

¼ teaspoon freshly ground black pepper

Oil or cooking spray

1 large egg

4 (4-ounce) boneless, skinless chicken breasts

Preheat the oven to 375° F. In a small bowl, combine the bread crumbs, Parmesan cheese, sesame seeds, oregano, tarragon, thyme, lemon rind, sea salt, and pepper. In another small bowl, beat the egg with 1 tablespoon of water and the lemon juice.

Lightly grease a baking pan with oil or cooking spray. Dip each chicken breast in the egg, then in the bread crumbs. Place the coated chicken in the prepared baking pan. Bake for 40 minutes, or until the chicken is golden brown and cooked through.

NUTRITIONAL INFORMATION PER SERVING:

240 calories · 32g protein · 14g carbohydrates · 2g fiber · 7g fat · 1g saturated fat · 257mg sodium

TURKEY MEATBALLS

Turkey meatballs are a great meal with tomato sauce, whole wheat pasta, and a side salad, or inside a sandwich or pita pocket. You can make a batch to freeze until you are ready to use them. *4 servings (2 meatballs per serving)*

1 pound ground lean turkey (7% fat)

2 green onions, chopped

1 large egg, beaten

2 cloves garlic, minced

1 teaspoon dried oregano

1 teaspoon dried basil

1 tablespoon ketchup

1 cup whole wheat bread crumbs,
   fresh or dried

1 tablespoon olive oil

1 tablespoon grated Parmesan cheese

Preheat the oven to 375° F. Line a baking pan with parchment paper or foil. In a large bowl, mix the turkey with the green onion, egg, garlic, oregano, basil, and ketchup, combining with clean hands. (And be sure to clean hands thoroughly after working with raw meat.) Gradually pour in the bread crumbs and continue mixing until all ingredients are combined.

Form the mixture into eight 1-inch balls and place in the prepared baking pan. Brush each meatball lightly with the oil and sprinkle with the cheese. Bake for 20 minutes, or until brown and cooked through.

NUTRITIONAL INFORMATION PER SERVING:

221 calories · 32g protein · 9g carbohydrates · 1g fiber · 6g fat · 1g saturated fat · 298mg sodium

TURKEY MEAT LOAF

This is a great make-ahead dish to cut into serving-size pieces and store in the fridge or the freezer. Any leftovers make a tasty sandwich on whole wheat bread. *4 servings*

Oil or cooking spray

1½ pounds lean ground turkey (7% fat)

1 large egg

½ packet dry onion soup mix

½ cup chopped red bell pepper

¼ cup rolled oats

1 tablespoon ketchup

Pinch of freshly ground black pepper

Preheat the oven to 350° F. Lightly grease a 9 × 5 × 3-inch loaf pan with oil or cooking spray. In a large bowl, mix the ground turkey and egg until well combined, and blend in the dry soup mix, red pepper, oats, ketchup, and pepper. Turn the mixture into the prepared loaf pan, tamp down, and bake for 45 to 60 minutes, or until cooked through.

239 calories · 43g protein · 6g carbohydrates · 1g fiber · 4g fat · 1g saturated fat · 572mg sodium

MOM'S TURKEY VEGETABLE CHILI

Mom makes the best chili, and hers is even better the next day. If you like, divide it into individual containers and freeze for easy meals later in the month. Many companies make organic ketchup, so you can have the great taste without the high-fructose corn syrup, food coloring, additives, and preservatives. The same goes for Worcestershire sauce (Annie's Naturals is one of my favorites). Remember to read the ingredients and buy the product with the fewest additives.

4 servings

3 tablespoons olive oil
1 clove garlic, finely chopped
8 ounces lean ground turkey (7% fat)
1 tablespoon chopped fresh basil
1 tablespoon dried oregano
1 red bell pepper, diced
1 yellow bell pepper, diced
1 large onion, diced
1 cup chopped celery
1 cup chopped carrots
1 cup chopped zucchini

1 (19-ounce) can bean medley
   containing navy beans, lima beans,
   kidney beans, and chickpeas
1 (12-ounce) can corn kernels, or
   12 ounces frozen corn
1 (28-ounce) can diced tomatoes
   (no added salt or sugar)
4 tablespoons Worcestershire sauce
¼ cup organic ketchup
1 tablespoon chili powder
½ tablespoon ground cumin

In a large skillet, heat the oil over medium heat. Sauté the garlic for 2 to 3 minutes, or until it begins to brown. Add the ground turkey, basil, and oregano and continue to cook about 10 minutes, until the turkey is golden brown.

In a large saucepan, combine the turkey mixture with the red and yellow peppers, onion, celery, carrots, zucchini, beans, corn, tomatoes, Worcestershire sauce, ketchup, chili powder, and cumin. Bring to a boil over medium heat. Reduce heat to low and simmer, covered, for 30 to 45 minutes, or until the vegetables are tender. Stir the chili occasionally as it cooks so it does not stick to the saucepan.

NUTRITIONAL INFORMATION PER SERVING:

464 calories • 30g protein • 70g carbohydrates • 12g fiber • 8g fat • 1g saturated fat • 745mg sodium

⭐ BROILED LEMON-GARLIC SEA BASS

When you don't have time to marinate fish, you can still add a great zesty flavor with lemon juice, garlic, and lemon pepper seasoning. *2 servings*

Cooking spray or 1 teaspoon olive oil
2 (4-ounce) sea bass fillets
1 tablespoon freshly squeezed lemon juice
1 clove garlic, minced
¼ teaspoon lemon pepper (no sodium)
¼ teaspoon freshly ground black pepper

Preheat the broiler with the rack positioned 4 inches from the heat source. Lightly spray a baking pan with cooking spray or coat with a teaspoon of olive oil. Place the fillets in the pan. Sprinkle the lemon juice, garlic, lemon pepper, and pepper over the fillets. Broil for 8 to 10 minutes, or until the fish is opaque. Serve immediately.

NUTRITIONAL INFORMATION PER SERVING:

141 calories • 27g protein • 2g carbohydrates • 3g fat • 1g saturated fat • 94mg sodium

HALIBUT WITH MANGO SALSA

Halibut is a cold-water fish that is packed with healthy fish oils and protein. It is a bit denser than some of the other fish so you will definitely feel satisfied when you are finished eating. The mango salsa can be served with chicken, salmon, trout, sole, or turkey. *2 servings*

1 large ripe mango, peeled and diced
½ small red bell pepper, seeded and diced
1 medium tomato, seeded and diced
1 whole green onion, chopped
2 tablespoons minced fresh ginger
1 clove garlic, minced

Juice of 1 lime
3 tablespoons chopped cilantro
2 (6-ounce) halibut fillets
¼ teaspoon sea salt or Himalayan salt
¼ teaspoon freshly ground black pepper

Preheat oven to 350° F. In a medium bowl, combine the mango, red pepper, tomato, green onion, ginger, garlic, lime juice, and cilantro. Mix well, cover, and refrigerate until ready to serve.

Season the fish fillets lightly with sea salt or Himalayan salt and pepper. Place in a nonstick baking dish. Bake for 10 to 12 minutes, or until flesh is white and opaque. Drizzle the mango salsa over the fish and serve immediately.

NUTRITIONAL INFORMATION PER SERVING:

357 calories • 46g protein • 29g carbohydrates • 4g fiber • 5g fat • 416mg sodium

BAKED TROUT

Baked trout is a light, healthy meal that is easy to prepare. To add variety to any fish or meat, try different-flavored salsas such as mango, tomato, melon, tropical fruit, or avocado. *2 servings*

2 (4-ounce) trout fillets
1½ tablespoons freshly squeezed lime
    juice

1 medium tomato, chopped
½ medium onion, chopped
1½ tablespoons chopped cilantro

1 teaspoon olive oil

¼ teaspoon freshly ground black pepper

¼ teaspoon sea salt or Himalayan salt

¼ teaspoon crushed red pepper

Juice of 1 lemon

Preheat the oven to 350° F. Rinse the fish fillets, pat dry with paper towels, and place in a baking dish large enough to hold the fillets so they don't overlap. In a medium bowl, mix together the lime juice, tomato, onion, cilantro, olive oil, pepper, salt, and crushed red pepper, then pour the mixture over the fish. Bake for 15 to 20 minutes, or until the fish is fork-tender. Remove fish to a warm platter or individual plates, sprinkle with fresh lemon juice, and serve.

NUTRITIONAL INFORMATION PER SERVING:

225 calories · 28g protein · 4g carbohydrates · 1g fiber · 10g fat · 3g saturated fat · 242mg sodium

★ BAKED ROMANO WILD TROUT

Wild trout is a cold-water fish that is packed with protein and omega-3 fatty acids, also known as healthy fish oils. Romano cheese adds an unexpected flavor when combined with Italian-style bread crumbs. The nutritional information is provided for the Italian-style bread crumbs.

4 servings

¾ cup Italian-style or plain whole wheat
   bread crumbs

2 tablespoons garlic powder

8 tablespoons grated Romano cheese

⅓ cup freshly squeezed lemon juice
   (or more as needed)

4 (4-ounce) wild trout fillets, rinsed and
   patted dry

4 tablespoons chopped parsley

Preheat the oven to 375° F. In a large bowl, combine the bread crumbs, garlic powder, Romano cheese, and enough lemon juice to form a paste.

   Cut a piece of parchment paper large enough to loosely enclose one trout fillet. Place a fillet on the parchment paper and spread ¼ of the paste evenly on top. Sprinkle with 1 tablespoon of parsley.

Fold the parchment paper to enclose the trout loosely and tuck the ends underneath, creating a sealed pocket. Repeat this process with the remaining fillets. Place on a baking sheet and bake for 10 to 12 minutes, or until the center of the fish is opaque.

NUTRITIONAL INFORMATION PER SERVING:

312 calories • 34g protein • 20g carbohydrates • 1g fiber • 11g fat • 4g saturated fat • 587mg sodium

BROILED HONEY-MUSTARD SALMON

Honey mustard is traditionally a great flavoring for chicken but it also adds zest to salmon.

1 serving

2 teaspoons Dijon mustard
1 tablespoon honey
1 (4-ounce) wild salmon fillet, skin removed
1 teaspoon freshly ground black pepper
Juice of ½ lemon

Preheat the broiler. Combine the mustard and honey and stir until well mixed and set aside. Sprinkle both sides of the salmon with the ground pepper and lightly coat one side of the fillet with the honey mustard. Place the fillet honey side up on a nonstick baking sheet and broil for 5 minutes on each side, or until salmon is opaque and light pink. Sprinkle with fresh lemon juice and serve.

NUTRITIONAL INFORMATION PER SERVING:

281 calories • 29g protein • 15g carbohydrates • 9g fat • 1g saturated fat • 305mg sodium • 0g fiber

POACHED WILD SALMON

Poaching is one of the best ways to cook fish so that you keep some of the healthy oils. Unfortunately, healthy oils are very sensitive to light, oxygen, and heat, and they are easily destroyed. Udo Erasmus, Ph.D., a pioneer in the study of healthy fats, claims that it is best to eat fish raw (sushi- or sashimi-style) to preserve the healthy fats; but if you must cook your fish, then poaching with the skin on is the best method. To be sure you get your daily dose of healthy oils, it may be best to take a supplement. Author and health expert Dr. Joseph Mercola recommends Carlson's fish oil supplement. You can read more on his Web site, www.mercola.com.

2 servings

½ onion, thinly sliced

1 lemon, thinly sliced

¼ teaspoon sea salt

¼ teaspoon whole peppercorns

1 sprig dill, or ¼ teaspoon dried dill weed

1 sprig parsley

2 (4-ounce) wild salmon fillets or
  salmon steaks

In a large skillet, combine 2½ cups water with the onion, lemon, sea salt, peppercorns, dill, and parsley over high heat and bring to a boil. Once boiling, reduce the heat to medium, cover, and let simmer for 10 minutes.

Add the salmon, cover, and continue to simmer for 5 minutes (a little longer for fillets or steaks that are thicker than ½ inch), or until fish flakes easily with a fork. Lift the fillets from the pan with a spatula, discard the residue, and serve.

NUTRITIONAL INFORMATION PER SERVING:

226 calories · 24g protein · 6g carbohydrates · 1g fiber · 9g fat · 1g saturated fat · 50mg sodium

TOFU VEGETABLE STIR-FRY

Tofu is very easy to digest and an excellent alternative source of protein if you don't want to eat meat. If you're short on time, replace the fresh vegetables with a package of frozen precut stir-fry vegetables, which offer the same nutritional value. You can use a store-bought Asian marinade or teriyaki sauce in place of the brown sauce; just make sure to read the labels and choose healthy organic marinades that are low in sugar, sodium, and calories. *2 servings*

1 tablespoon grapeseed oil

½ medium onion, sliced

1 tablespoon grated fresh ginger

2 cloves garlic, minced

8 ounces firm or extra-firm tofu, drained and diced into bite-size pieces

2 tablespoons rice wine vinegar

1 tablespoon honey or sugar

1 tablespoon low-sodium soy sauce

1 teaspoon cornstarch mixed with 1 tablespoon cold water

2 cups chopped broccoli

1 red bell pepper, thinly sliced

½ cup thinly sliced jicama

1½ cups mushrooms, sliced

½ tablespoon toasted sesame seed

1 cup steamed brown rice

In a large wok or skillet, heat the oil over medium heat. Stir in the onion and cook for 1 minute, or until clear and lightly browned. Add the ginger and garlic and cook for 30 seconds. Stir in the tofu and cook about 4 minutes, until golden brown on all sides. Remove the tofu mixture from the wok and drain on a paper towel.

In a small saucepan, combine ¼ cup of water with the rice wine vinegar, honey or sugar, and soy sauce and bring to a simmer. Cook for 2 minutes and stir in the cornstarch mixture. Simmer until the sauce thickens and set aside.

Add the broccoli, pepper, jicama, and mushrooms to the same wok or skillet. If necessary, add a teaspoon of oil. Sauté the vegetables for 2 minutes over medium heat, add the sauce, and cover and cook for 1 to 2 minutes, until the broccoli is bright green and tender-crisp. Add the tofu and sesame seed and toss to coat evenly. Heat thoroughly and serve with steamed brown rice.

NUTRITIONAL INFORMATION PER SERVING:

454 calories · 21g protein · 65g carbohydrates · 16g fiber · 15g fat · 2g saturated fat · 336mg sodium

TURKEY LASAGNA

Here's a recipe that's a healthy alternative to lasagna that uses ground beef. This turkey version is delicious and only has 4 grams of saturated fat per serving, which comes from the low-fat mozzarella cheese. *6 servings*

9 whole wheat lasagna noodles

1 tablespoon olive oil

1 pound lean ground turkey (7% fat)

1 medium onion, chopped (about ½ cup)

2 cloves garlic, finely chopped

4 cups marinara pasta sauce or your favorite flavor

6 cups fresh spinach

5 basil leaves

4 cups low-fat cottage cheese

1½ cups shredded low-fat mozzarella cheese

4 tablespoons grated Reggiano Parmigiano cheese

Preheat the oven to 350° F.

Bring 6 quarts of lightly salted water to a boil, add the noodles, and cook until they are al dente, soft but still firm. Drain in a colander, toss with 1 tablespoon of olive oil, and lay flat to cool on a cookie sheet to prevent sticking.

Heat a large nonstick skillet over medium heat and add the ground turkey, onion, and garlic and cook about 10 minutes, until the turkey is browned. Drain excess fat. Mix in the marinara sauce until it is well combined with the turkey. Reduce the heat to low and simmer for 5 minutes.

In a double boiler with a steamer top, steam the spinach for about 3 minutes, or until wilted. Remove from heat and set aside to cool.

Spoon a thin layer of the sauce into an ungreased 10 × 8 × 2-inch baking dish and arrange a single layer of noodles (about three; cut to fit if necessary) on top, slightly overlapping. Spread about one-third of the turkey sauce over the noodles. Cover the turkey with the basil leaves and all of the spinach. Cover the spinach with half of the cottage cheese. Sprinkle one-third of the mozzarella on top.

Continue layering with three more lasagna noodles, one-third of the turkey sauce, the remaining cottage cheese, and one-third of the mozzarella. Finish with the last layer of noodles, the remaining turkey sauce, and the remaining mozzarella cheese. Sprinkle the grated Reggiano Parmigiano on top.

Cover with foil and bake for 30 to 40 minutes, or until bubbling. Remove the foil and bake for 5 minutes more, or until the cheese is golden.

NUTRITIONAL INFORMATION PER SERVING:

429 calories · 54g protein · 44g carbohydrates · 8g fiber · 14g fat · 4g saturated fat · 831mg sodium

QUICK-AND-EASY TURKEY TOMATO PENNE

Whole wheat and gluten-free brown rice pastas are healthier options than the versions made from white flour. These are not only less refined but, because of the higher fiber content, they also make you feel fuller longer without eating as much. *4 servings*

SAUCE
12 ounces lean ground turkey (7% fat)
2 teaspoons chopped fresh basil pasta (for each serving)
2 teaspoons chopped fresh oregano
1 (16-ounce) can low-sodium tomato pasta sauce (Muir Glen is a popular organic pasta sauce brand with several different flavors.)

PASTA
1 cup uncooked whole wheat penne pasta (for each serving)

In a large heavy nonstick skillet, cook the turkey, basil, and oregano over medium heat for about 10 minutes, until the turkey is cooked through. Drain excess fat. Add the tomato sauce and let simmer, covered, over low heat while you prepare the pasta. Cook the penne according to the package directions, using about 2 cups of water for every cup of dry pasta, and bring to a boil in a medium saucepan. Drain the pasta and return to the saucepan. Toss the pasta and the warm sauce to coat evenly and serve immediately. You can also store individual portions in microwave-safe containers to reheat for "brown bag" lunches, but be sure to keep the food cool until you are ready to eat.

NUTRITIONAL INFORMATION PER SERVING:

362 calories · 31g protein · 55g carbohydrates · 6g fiber · 3g fat · 1g saturated fat · 73mg sodium

APPLE CRISP

This is a great dessert for the whole family. You can add a scoop of low-fat frozen yogurt, but make sure you factor in the additional calories to your daily total (see chart, pp. 246–254). *8 servings*

½ cup whole wheat flour
¾ cup old-fashioned rolled oats
½ cup packed light brown sugar
1 teaspoon ground cinnamon
½ teaspoon ground nutmeg

¼ cup chilled organic unsalted butter
Cooking spray
6 cups peeled, cored, and chopped
   Granny Smith apples

Preheat the oven to 375° F. In a medium bowl, combine the flour, oats, ¼ cup of the brown sugar, ½ teaspoon of the cinnamon, and the nutmeg. Cut in the butter with a pastry blender or two knives until the mixture resembles coarse meal.

Coat a 13 × 9 × 2-inch baking pan with cooking spray. In a medium bowl, mix the apples with the remaining brown sugar and the remaining cinnamon and place them in the prepared baking dish. Top with the oat mixture. Bake for 30 minutes, or until the apples are tender.

NUTRITIONAL INFORMATION PER SERVING:

226 calories · 4g protein · 39g carbohydrates · 4g fiber · 7g fat · 4g saturated fat · 0mg sodium

CHEF RONNDA'S CARAMELIZED APPLES

If you love apple pie, then you will love these caramelized apples. They are actually very light— and delicious! *1 serving*

1 green apple, peeled, cored, and thickly
   sliced
1 teaspoon chopped fresh thyme
½ teaspoon vanilla extract

2 tablespoons maple syrup
½ teaspoon freshly squeezed lemon juice
1 tablespoon olive oil
1 tablespoon slivered almonds

In a large bowl, toss the apples, thyme, vanilla, maple syrup, and lemon juice until the apples are completely coated.

In a large skillet, heat the oil over medium heat and add the apples. Cook for 3 to 5 minutes, until the apples are slightly brown but still firm, stirring frequently. Remove from heat and serve garnished with slivered almonds.

NUTRITIONAL INFORMATION PER SERVING:

274 calories · 1g protein · 36g carbohydrates · 2g fiber · 15g fat · 2g saturated fat · 3mg sodium

APPLE WALNUT DESSERT

Simple yet satisfying! Greek yogurt has a thicker consistency than most others, similar to sour cream, which makes it ideal for this dessert. *1 serving*

1 apple, peeled, cored, and chopped into pieces
3 ounces low-fat plain or Greek yogurt
1 tablespoon chopped walnuts
½ teaspoon ground cinnamon

Place the chopped apple in a small bowl and top with the yogurt, walnuts, and cinnamon.

NUTRITIONAL INFORMATION PER SERVING:

179 calories · 6g protein · 30g carbohydrates · 3g fiber · 6g fat · 0g saturated fat · 0mg sodium

DARK CHOCOLATE–COVERED STRAWBERRIES

Everyone loves chocolate and strawberries. I have chosen dark chocolate for this recipe because it has a phytonutrient called epicatechin, which is a particularly active member of a group of compounds called plant flavonoids. Flavonoids help keep cholesterol from gathering in blood vessels, reduce the risk of blood clots, and slow down the immune responses that lead to clogged arteries. Choose an organic dark chocolate, and always read the ingredients to make sure there aren't any added preservatives or chemicals. *4 servings*

12 toothpicks for dipping
16 fresh large strawberries
5 ounces dark chocolate (chips or bar)
1 tablespoon canola oil

Insert a toothpick into the top of each strawberry. Cover a cookie sheet with waxed paper.

In the top of a double boiler, melt the chocolate with the oil until smooth, stirring occasionally. Holding the berries by the toothpicks, dip them halfway into the chocolate, making sure not to completely cover them.

Place the strawberries on the prepared cookie sheet and chill in the refrigerator until ready to serve.

NUTRITIONAL INFORMATION PER SERVING (4 STRAWBERRIES):

225 calories • 2g protein • 26g carbohydrates • 3g fiber • 12g fat • 7g saturated fat • 6mg sodium

⭐ BLUEBERRY MINI CAKES

These cakes are so scrumptious you'll be tempted to eat more than one, but they keep well in the refrigerator or freezer so don't give in. These little treats deliver a good dose of fiber, and you'll feel satisfied with just one. They make a convenient snack, too. *Makes 12 cakes*

1½ cups wheat bran
1 cup low-fat milk
½ cup applesauce
1 large egg
¾ cup packed light brown sugar
½ teaspoon vanilla extract

1 cup whole wheat flour
1 teaspoon baking soda
1 teaspoon baking powder
½ teaspoon salt
1 cup fresh or frozen blueberries

Preheat the oven to 375° F. Line a 12-cup muffin pan with paper muffin cups.

In a medium bowl, combine the wheat bran and milk and let stand for 10 minutes. In a separate large bowl, mix the applesauce, egg, brown sugar, and vanilla. Beat in the bran mixture until all of the ingredients are well combined.

Sift together the whole wheat flour, baking soda, baking powder, and salt. Stir dry ingredients into the bran mixture until just blended. Mix in the blueberries. Scoop the batter into the muffin cups and bake for 15 to 20 minutes, or until cakes are high and browned on top. You can test for doneness with a toothpick that should come away clean.

NUTRITIONAL INFORMATION PER CAKE:

131 calories · 4g protein · 30g carbohydrates · 5g fiber · 1g fat · 0g saturated fat · 223mg sodium

CHEF RONNDA'S ALMOND RICOTTA CHEESECAKE

This recipe is silky and satisfying, smooth and not overly sweet. The nutritional information provided is for skim ricotta cheese. If you use part-skim ricotta cheese, you will have to make small changes to your nutritional counts (see chart, pp. 246–254). *8 servings*

3 cups skim or part-skim ricotta cheese
2 large eggs
2 teaspoons vanilla extract
¾ cup sliced toasted almonds
2 teaspoons almond extract
4 teaspoons ground cinnamon
¾ cup maple syrup

Preheat the oven to 350° F. In a large bowl, combine all of the ingredients until well blended. Pour the batter into a 9-inch nonstick baking pan. Bake for 30 to 40 minutes, until the cake is firm. Remove from the oven, and allow to set for about 1 hour, or until the cake is completely cool, before serving.

NUTRITIONAL INFORMATION PER SERVING:

279 calories · 14g protein · 28g carbohydrates · 2g fiber · 13g fat · 5g saturated fat · 115mg sodium

CALIFORNIA FRUIT SALAD

Fresh fruit is refreshing and light. The coconut flakes are a great added touch that creates a little extra sweetness. *2 servings*

1 cup fresh pineapple chunks or canned in natural juices, drained

1 cup sliced strawberries

½ cup blueberries

1 orange, peeled, sectioned, and cut into pieces

1 apple, peeled, cored, and chopped

2 tablespoons raw coconut flakes

In a large bowl, mix all the fruits together gently. Turn out into individual serving bowls, sprinkle with coconut flakes, and serve.

NUTRITIONAL INFORMATION PER SERVING:

172 calories · 2g protein · 40g carbohydrates · 8g fiber · 2g fat · 2g saturated fat · 0mg sodium

OATMEAL RAISIN COOKIES

This recipe calls for whole wheat flour instead of white to make the cookie higher in fiber and turn it into a healthy snack or dessert. *Makes 30 cookies*

½ cup packed light brown sugar

1 large egg

1 egg white

¾ cup applesauce

1 teaspoon vanilla extract

1½ cups whole wheat flour

1 teaspoon baking soda

1½ teaspoons ground cinnamon

¼ teaspoon ground nutmeg

1½ cups old-fashioned rolled oats

¾ cup raisins

½ cup walnuts, coarsely chopped

Cooking spray or parchment paper

Preheat the oven to 350° F. In a large bowl, mix the brown sugar, egg, egg white, applesauce, and vanilla until combined. Add the flour, baking soda, cinnamon, and nutmeg and stir until well combined. Stir in the oats, raisins, and walnuts.

Prepare two baking sheets by either spraying with cooking spray or lining with parchment paper. Drop the dough by heaping teaspoonfuls onto the prepared sheets and flatten with a fork. Bake for 8 to10 minutes, then transfer to a wire rack to cool.

NUTRITIONAL INFORMATION PER COOKIE:

94 calories · 3g protein · 17g carbohydrates · 2g fiber · 2g fat · 48mg sodium · 0g saturated fat

CHEF RONNDA'S SEXY STRAWBERRY WALNUT DESSERT

There's a touch of added sweetness from the maple syrup, which is loaded with manganese and zinc, making this a healthy alternative to a high-sugar dessert. *4 servings*

- 4 cups fresh or frozen strawberries (thawed), sliced
- 8 tablespoons maple syrup
- 2 teaspoons vanilla extract
- 4 tablespoons finely chopped walnuts, toasted

Preheat the oven to 350° F. In a medium bowl, toss the strawberries with the maple syrup and vanilla. Spread in a single layer on a baking sheet. Bake for 20 minutes, or until soft and tender. You can toast the chopped walnuts at the same time in the oven. Spread them on a separate baking sheet and place on a different rack for 5 to 8 minutes. Serve the berries warm or cool, topped with the walnuts.

NUTRITIONAL INFORMATION PER SERVING:

179 calories · 3g protein · 34g carbohydrates · 4g fiber · 1g fat · 3mg sodium · 0g saturated fat

INDIVIDUAL FOOD COUNTS

Food Name	SERVING SIZE	CALORIES	PROTEIN GMS	CARB. GMS	FIBER GMS	FAT GMS	SAT. FAT GMS	SODIUM MGS
Acorn squash	1 medium	167	3.3	43	13	0.5		15

Almonds
  Sliced, toasted
  Whole
	
	¾ cup
	23
		
		399
		164
			
			14.7
			6
				
				13.6
				5.6
					
					8.1
						
						34.9
						14.4
							
							2.7
							1.1	

Apple	1 medium	80	0.4	21.3	3.7	0.3		2
Apple cider	2 cups	191		50				
Applesauce	¼ cup	52		14	1.5			
Asian marinade	2 Tbsp	60		12		1		680
Asparagus	12 oz	68	7.5	13.2	7.2	0.4		
Avocado	1 oz	45	0.6	2.4	1.9	4.2	0.6	2
Bagel, whole wheat	1 medium-size	150	6.2	32	5.3	1		300
Baking powder	1 tsp	5		2.3	0.1			5
Baking soda	1 tsp							1,259
Balsamic salad dressing, fat-free	2 Tbsp	25		6				350
Balsamic vinegar	2 Tbsp	20		4				10
Banana	1 medium	105	1.3	27	3.1	0.4		1
Bean medley (navy, lima, kidney, chickpeas)	19-oz can	635	41.5	107.9	20.8	4.2		830
Berries, mixed (blueberries, raspberries, blackberries)	½ cup	45	1	11	3.4	0.6		1.71
Black beans, rinsed and drained	14 oz	457	31.7	77.4	17.6	3.5	1.8	1,119
Black olives	8–10	25		1		2	2	110
Blueberries	1 cup	83	1.1	20	4	0.5		
Bread, 100% whole wheat	1 slice	78	3	14.8	2.2	1		105

Food Name	SERVING SIZE	CALORIES	PROTEIN GMS	CARB. GMS	FIBER GMS	FAT GMS	SAT. FAT GMS	SODIUM MGS
Bread crumbs, fresh or dried	1 cup	156	6	29.6	4.4	2		210
Broccoli	2 cups	62	5.1	12.1	4.7			60
Brown rice, cooked	½ cup	108	2.5	22.4	1.8	0.9		5
Brown-rice cake, salt-free	1	70	1	16	0.5			
Brussels sprouts	1 lb	225	15.9	44.3	16.2	3.1		
Burger bun, sprouted grain	1	170	9	32	6	1.5	1.5	180
Butter, unsalted	1 Tbsp	100				11	7	0
Butternut squash	1 medium (about 3 lbs)	328	7.4	86		1		
Cabbage, shredded	1 cup	21	1.3	5		0.1		16
Caesar salad dressing	2 Tbsp	120	2	2		11	1.5	190
Canola oil	1 Tbsp	108				12	1	80
Cantaloupe	½ medium	94	2.3	22.5	2.5	0.5	0.1	44
Carrots								
Baby	1 cup	50	1.2	11.2	4.4	0.4		
Chopped	1 cup	52	1.2	12.3	3.6	0.3		88
Celery, chopped	1 cup	17	0.8	3.6	1.9	0.2		96
Cheese								
Monterey Jack, reduced-fat shredded	¼ cup	80	8	1		5		180
Mozzarella, low-fat shredded	1½ cups	360	42	6		30	18	960
String, organic low-fat or part-skim	1 string	60	6	1		3.5	2.5	110

Food Name	SERVING SIZE	CALORIES	PROTEIN GMS	CARB. GMS	FIBER GMS	FAT GMS	SAT. FAT GMS	SODIUM MGS
Chicken breast, boneless, skinless	6 oz 4 oz	183 120	35 26			3.9 1.5	1.1	443 75
Chicken broth, low-sodium, nonfat	1 cup	25	4	1				140
Chickpeas (garbanzo beans), canned	¼ cup	68	2.8	12.8	2.5	0.6		170
Chocolate, organic dark (chips or bar)	1 oz	144	1.6	17.3	1.4	9.3	5	
Cinnamon, ground	1 tsp	6		1.8	1.2			
Coconut flakes, raw	0.3 oz (2 Tbsp)	34	0.3	1.5	1	3.2	2.9	
Corn niblets (canned or frozen)	12 oz	269	8.2	66.1	6.8	1.7		10
Cornstarch	1 Tbsp	54		13	0.1			
Cottage cheese, low sodium, low-fat	½ cup 1 cup	81 160	14 28	3 4		1 2		14 28
Crackers, low-fat whole wheat	Approx. 5 crackers	116	4.5	19	3.5			213
Cranberries, dried	¼ cup	90.75		24	2.4			
Cream cheese, low-fat	2 Tbsp	69	3.2	2	5.3	3		88
Cucumber, diced	½ medium	12	0.6	2.2	0.7	0.2		2
Cumin, ground	1½ tsp	12	0.6	1.4	0.3	0.7		
Curry powder	¼ tsp	7	0.3	1.2	0.7	0.3		
Egg	1	77	6			5	1.6	139
Egg whites	3 4 ¾ cup	49 66 91	10 14 19	1 1 1.8				162 219 298
Feta cheese, reduced-fat, crumbled	¼ cup	76	7.6			4.9	3.3	

Food Name	SERVING SIZE	CALORIES	PROTEIN GMS	CARB. GMS	FIBER GMS	FAT GMS	SAT. FAT GMS	SODIUM MGS
Flaxseed oil, organic	1 Tbsp	120				13.6 (11.3 healthy omega-3 and omega-6 unsatu-rated fats)	1.3	
Flour, whole wheat	½ cup	203	8.2	43.5	7.3	1.1	0.2	3
Garlic, minced	1 clove	4		1				
Garlic powder	2 Tbsp	56	2.8	12.2	1.7	0.1		4
Ginger, minced fresh	2 Tbsp	37	1	7.6	1.4	0.6		3
Granola, low-fat	¼ cup	115	3	22.7	2	1.5		5
Grapefruit, pink	½	37		9	1.5			
Grapeseed oil	1 Tbsp	120				13.6	1.3	
Greek salad dressing, organic	4 Tbsp	111	1	2		11		350
Greek yogurt, nonfat	1 cup (8 oz)	121	22.7	9.1		0		167
Green beans	12 oz	106	6.2	24.3	11.6	0.4		20
Green onions	2 medium	9.6	1	2.2	1			4.8
Guacamole	4 Tbsp	89	1.8	5.3		8	4.4	
Half-and-half	1 oz	39	1	1.29		3.45	2.15	12.2
Halibut fillet	6 oz	241	44.1			4		120
Honey	1 Tbsp	64		17.3				
Hot sauce	1 tsp							124
Hummus, organic	4 Tbsp	93	4.4	8	3.4	5.4		212
Jalapeño pepper	1 small	4.2	0.2	0.8	0.4			
Jam, all fruit, blueberry	1½ Tbsp	36		9	0.5			

Food Name	SERVING SIZE	CALORIES	PROTEIN GMS	CARB. GMS	FIBER GMS	FAT GMS	SAT. FAT GMS	SODIUM MGS
Jicama, thinly sliced	½ cup	125	2.4	29.1	16.1			13
Ketchup, organic	¼ cup	68		16.7				635
	1 Tbsp	15		3				150
Lamb chop, trimmed of fat	5 oz	287	38			13.8	5	94
Lasagna noodles, whole wheat	9	810	36	153	31.5	6.8		23
	1	90	4	17	3.5	0.8		2.6
Lemon juice	Juice of 1	15		5.3	0.2			1
Lemon pepper herb seasoning, no sodium								
Lettuce, baby organic green	½ cup	4	0.5	0.7	0.5			2
Lime juice	Juice of 1	10		3.2	0.2			
Mandarin oranges	2 small	74	1.1	18.7	2.5	0.4		3
Mango	½ of 1 or 3 slices	67		17.5	2			2
	1 large ripe	135	1.1	35.2	3.7	0.6		4
Maple syrup	1 Tbsp	52		13				
Mayonnaise, organic light	2 Tbsp	72		2		7		220
Milk, low-fat	1 cup	100	8	12		2.5	1.5	125
Mixed greens	1 cup	7	0.6	1.4	1			
Mushrooms	¼ cup (1.5 oz)	9	1.3	1.4	0.4			
Mustard	3 tsp	9.9	0.6			0.4		168
Mustard, Dijon	2 tsp	10	0.5	2				240
Nutmeg	½ tsp	6	0.1	0.5	0.2	0.4	0.3	
Oatmeal Cooked	1½ cups	218	9	38	6	3.6	0.6	
Uncooked	¼ cup	72	3	12	2	1		

Food Name	SERVING SIZE	CALORIES	PROTEIN GMS	CARB. GMS	FIBER GMS	FAT GMS	SAT. FAT GMS	SODIUM MGS
Olive oil	½ Tbsp	59.7				6.8	1	
Onion								
Chopped	¼ cup	10		3.5				
Whole	1 large	63	1.4	15.2	2.1	0.1		5
Onion soup mix*	½ packet, dry	59	1.5	11.8	1.3	1		1,566
Orange juice	½ cup	56	1	12.9	0.2			
Pancake								
Buckwheat mix*	When prepared, 2 6-inch pancakes	234	8	36	6	2	2	580
Dry blue corn mix*	⅓ cup	160	5	30	5	1.5		270
Parmesan cheese	1 tsp	10	1			0.7		42
	1 Tbsp	22	2			1.4	0.8	70
Parmigiano Reggiano cheese, grated	4 Tbsp	80	8			6	4	120
Parsley leaves	1 Tbsp	1		0.2	0.1			2
Pasta sauce, low-sodium tomato and basil	4 oz	40	2	9				20
Pear	1 medium	96	0.6	25.7	5.1	0.2		2
Penne pasta, whole wheat	1 cup	231	7.7	46.2	5.5	1.7		11
Pepper								
Green	1 medium	24	1	5.5	2	0.2		4
Red	1 medium	31	1.2	7.2	2.4			
Yellow	1 medium	50	1.9	11.8	1.7	0.4		4
Diced, red or yellow	¼ cup	10	0.4	2.2	0.7	0.1		1
Pineapple chunks	1 cup	74	0.8	19.6	2.2	0.2		
Pine nuts	2 oz	320	13	8	3	28	4.5	

*Varies by brand.

Food Name	SERVING SIZE	CALORIES	PROTEIN GMS	CARB. GMS	FIBER GMS	FAT GMS	SAT. FAT GMS	SODIUM MGS
Pineapple juice, unsweetened	⅓ cup	44	0.3	10.6	0.2	0.1		2
Pita, whole wheat organic	1	170	6.3	35.2	4.7	1.7	0.3	340
Pork tenderloin	4 oz	186	32			5.5	1.9	63.5
Potato	1 medium	161	4.4	37	3.8			
Potato, red	1 Tbsp	12		2.9				
Prosciutto di Parma, diced	1 oz	55	8			2.3	0.7	712
Raisins or currants	14	23		6.2	0.3			
Rapini	1 lb	144	16.7	13.6	12.2	2.3		245
Ricotta cheese, skim	1 cup	339	28	12.6		19.5		308
Romaine lettuce	5 cups	40	2.9	7.7	4.9	0.7		
Romano cheese, grated	8 Tbsp	160	16			12	8	680
Salmon, canned in water	6 oz	179	30			6	3	837
Salmon fillet, wild, skin removed	4 oz	207	28.9			9.2	1.4	64
Salsa	2 Tbsp	10		2				200
Salt	1 tsp							2,300
Scallions, diced	2	10	0.5	2.2		0.1		5
Sea bass fillets	4 oz	133.5	26.8			2.7	1.4	94
Sesame oil, dark	1 Tbsp	120				14	2	
Sesame seeds, toasted	½ Tbsp	24	0.7	1.1		2		
Shallots, minced	1 tsp	3.6		0.8				
Smoked salmon	3 oz (4 small slices)	100	16			3.7	0.8	500

Food Name	SERVING SIZE	CALORIES	PROTEIN GMS	CARB. GMS	FIBER GMS	FAT GMS	SAT. FAT GMS	SODIUM MGS
Sorbet, lemon	½ cup	140		35				
Soy nut butter	1 Tbsp	85	3.5	5	1.5	5.5		70
Soy sauce, low-sodium	1 Tbsp	10	0.9	1.5				600
Spinach, uncooked	2 cups	13	1.7	2.1	1.62			47
Squash, yellow summer, sliced	2	63	4.7	13.1	4.3	0.7	0.1	39
Steak, top sirloin, lean cut, from grass-fed cow with no hormones	4 oz	208	34.7				6.6	2.5	73
Stir-fry vegetables, frozen	2 cups	60	2	10	4			
Strawberries, sliced	½ cup	23		5	2			
Sugar	½ tsp 4 tsp	5 45		1.4 11.7				
Sweet potato	1 large	162	3.6	37.3	6			
Taco seasoning, low-sodium*	2 tsp	15		4				330
Teriyaki sauce*	2 Tbsp	60		12		1		680
Tofu, firm or extra-firm, drained	8 oz	230	23	5.8	2.9	11.5	1.4	
Tomato Diced, no-salt-added Cherry Roma	2 slices 28-oz can 4 8 13	10 125 14 29 455	0.4 6.3 0.5 1.1 13	2 25 3.1 6.3 91	0.5 6.3 1 1.5 13	 13		3 282 6 12 65
Tomato juice, no-salt-added	8 fl oz	41	1.8	10.3	1			24
Tortilla, whole wheat	1 6-inch	80	3	12	8	2		240

*Varies by brand.

Food Name	SERVING SIZE	CALORIES	PROTEIN GMS	CARB. GMS	FIBER GMS	FAT GMS	SAT. FAT GMS	SODIUM MGS
Trout, wild	4 oz	170	26			6.6	1.8	64
Tuna								
Canned in water	5.8 oz	191	42.1			1.4		558
Albacore canned in water	3 oz	105	22.4			1.5		374
Turkey								
Bacon	2 slices	70	4			5		360
Breast meat	2.5 oz	77	18	3				35
Lean ground	4 oz	160	22			8	2.5	85
Sandwich meat	4 thin slices	125	25.52			1.8	0.5	350
Sausage, low-fat	1 (90 grams)	130	14	2		6	2	400
Sausage patty	1 small (2–3 inches in diameter)	112	13			6	1.5	370
Vanilla extract	½ tsp	6		0.3				
Vegetable juice, low-sodium	8 oz	50	2	10	2			140
Vinegar								
Red wine								
Rice wine								
White wine								
Walnuts	1 oz or 14 halves	46	1.1	1	0.5	4.6		
Wheat bran	1½ cups	188	13.5	56.1	37.2	3.2		2
Wheat germ, toasted	⅛ cup	54	4.1	7	2.1	1.5		1
Whey protein, vanilla (depending on brand)	2 scoops	156	30	9		1		
Worcestershire sauce	4 Tbsp	40		10				920
Yogurt, plain, low-fat	1 8-oz cup	160	13	17		3.8	2.5	172
Zucchini, chopped	1 cup	20	1.5	4.2	1.4	0.2		

Part Five

YOU HAVE TO MOVE IT TO LOSE IT!

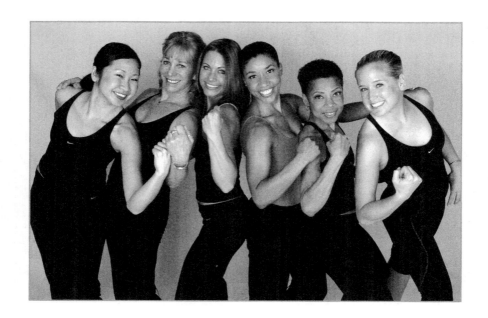

This section of the book is dedicated to exercise—and the specific exercises that you need to do to lose weight. Here, you'll discover the very foundations of effective exercise and why it's so important for you to not only know *what* to do but *how* to do it to get the best results.

By understanding the principles and fundamentals of effective fitness training, you will readily see what separates The Hollywood Trainer Weight-Loss Plan's exercise program from all the others.

I truly want to see you succeed and I know that some people just learn better by watching someone else do the exercises first. That's why I want to draw your attention to *The Hollywood Trainer Weight-Loss Plan Workout* DVD, which demonstrates every exercise in this book. If you do not already have this DVD, visit my Web site, www.thehollywoodtrainer.com, for more information.

18

WHAT DO I HAVE TO DO TO LOSE THIS WEIGHT?

That is the number one question I have been asked over the many years I've been involved in fitness. Most people point directly to their stomach and ask: "How can I get rid of the extra fat here?" The fact is, there is no magic pill, no quick-fix surgery, and no special celebrity diet that will work for everyone all of the time. To lose the weight, you have to adopt healthy habits through a holistic program that addresses your mind, body, and soul. Although this section of the book is dedicated specifically to the exercises required to lose weight and keep it off for good, it is important to review once again all seven steps of this program. Your success will come from the sum of all the steps.

1. You have to *accept that you must make a change*.
2. You have to *make a mental and spiritual change* in the way you think about yourself, eating, and exercise.
3. You have to *start exercising* and, more specifically, you have to do aerobic or cardiovascular training, resistance training, core training, and flexibility training.
4. You have to *eat foods that are wholesome and high quality* and decrease your portion sizes so you ingest fewer calories than you burn.

5. You have to *educate yourself about nutrition, exercise, and your body* so you can continue to make healthy choices for yourself and your family.

6. You need to *stay committed to and consistent about* positive thinking, exercising, healthy eating, and educating yourself.

7. You need to *build a supportive environment* so that when the going gets tough you have support from yourself, your faith, your friends, your workout buddy, and your family.

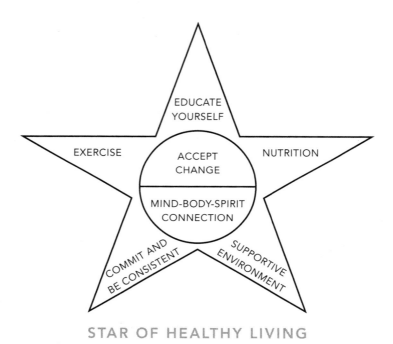

STAR OF HEALTHY LIVING

Every one of these steps is important, but exercise, which is the focus of this section, is a major component of the program. And to really understand how and why the Hollywood Trainer Weight-Loss Plan's exercise program works, you will want to read about the underlying principles and the fundamental components that are the foundations of my approach to fitness and well-being. Remember Step 5—Educate yourself! Educate yourself so that you'll get the best results because you'll understand why you do what you need to do, which will give you the motivation to keep doing it.

19

THE 6 ESSENTIAL PRINCIPLES
OF EXERCISE TRAINING

To maximize your results and minimize your risk of injury and setbacks, every good training regimen should be founded on basic principles that will produce results. The problem is that a lot of trainers, authors, and self-styled fitness gurus ignore these principles—to your detriment. Since I want you to be able to adopt exercise as a healthy daily habit, just like brushing your teeth and washing your face, I realize the importance of *explaining* how to guarantee results. When you were a kid, your mom told you to brush up and down, not side to side, or you wouldn't get your teeth really clean. The same theory applies to fitness: do it right and it will work. I know most of you have tried various exercise programs, lost a bit of weight at the beginning, and then become frustrated because your body stopped changing. Being unable to get past the "plateau" isn't your fault . . . it's because the *program has been poorly designed*. These six exercise training principles are the cornerstone of a good program design that will guarantee that you'll break through the plateau and maximize results:

1. *Individual Differences:* Every person is different, and each person's response to exercise will vary. A proper training program should take individual differences into account. I incorporate this principle by offering various levels of training in all of the daily

workout programs, so whether you are a beginner or intermediate student, there is a safe place for you to start and a challenging place toward which you can strive.

2. *Specificity:* To become better at a particular exercise or skill, you must perform that specific exercise or skill. In other words, to tone and strengthen your abdominals you have to include abdominal exercises in your program. To tone your thighs you have to include specific exercises for your thighs. If you want to improve your ability to jog, then you have to include jogging in your training. This principle also states that you should move from more general movements to more specific movements. This principle is the reason I added a specific Core Workout and drop sets in the circuits.

3. *Use/Disuse:* You have to move your muscles or they become soft and flabby. In simple terms, you've got to use it or you'll lose it! You must be committed and consistent to see results. Many people try to lose weight by working out just sporadically—when they feel like it—but they soon give up because they don't see results. Following a program consistently that has been designed for burning fat and reshaping your body will get you to your goals much faster and with a lot less frustration.

4. *Adaptation:* By repeating an exercise, the body adapts to the stress, and the skill becomes easier to perform. This also explains the need to continue to apply the principle of Overload to continue to see improvements in your physique.

5. *Overload:* A greater-than-normal load on the body is required to create change. If your body is already used to walking, then it is necessary to start incorporating an incline or jogging intervals. If your body is used to lifting 3-pound weights then you have to move up to 5-pounders to see results. The more you do, the more you become capable of doing. This is how all the training adaptations occur in exercise and training. The human body is an amazing machine. When you stress your body by lifting more weight than you are accustomed to, your body will react with physiological changes that will enable you to handle the stress the next time it occurs. This concept is the same in cardiovascular training relating to the heart, lungs, and endurance muscles. This is how people get stronger, bigger, and faster, and increase their physical fitness level. The Hollywood Trainer Weight-Loss Plan's exercise program provides several levels of intensity so your body can enjoy the benefits from the Overload principle.

6. *Progression:* There is an optimal level of overload that should be achieved, and an optimal time frame in which this overload should occur. Overload should not be increased too slowly or improvement is unlikely. If increased too rapidly, injury or

muscle damage may result. Therefore it's important that you start slowly and then progress to the next level as your body adapts to the exercise. That is why I have provided training logs and heart-rate monitoring in my program, so you can determine when to progress as your body adapts.

The six essential principles of exercise training give a theoretical framework to my program and help you understand why you need to do the things that are laid out in future chapters. But it is the four fundamental components of fitness—cardiorespiratory health, muscular strength, muscular endurance, and flexibility—that provide the means to put theory into action.

20

THE 4 FUNDAMENTALS OF FITNESS: CARDIORESPIRATORY HEALTH, MUSCULAR STRENGTH, MUSCULAR ENDURANCE, AND FLEXIBILITY

A multilevel weekly exercise program that incorporates all four components of fitness is the best workout for burning fat, losing weight, and reshaping your body. In Part 2 you conducted fitness tests for each one. A quick review of your Personal Fitness Profile will show in what areas you scored high and where you scored low. Now it's time to take a deeper look at how each component of fitness will help you lose weight, tone and define your muscles, increase your vitality, and keep you moving from morning until night.

CARDIORESPIRATORY HEALTH

Cardiorespiratory health is measured by your body's ability to get oxygen and blood to the working muscles. The term *cardiorespiratory fitness* is often interchanged with *cardiovascular* or *aerobic fitness, aerobics,* or simply *cardio.*

Remember the Rockport Fitness Walking Test (cardiorespiratory fitness test) that you did in your Personal Fitness Profile in Part 2? The purpose of that test was to determine your body's ability to get oxygen and blood to your working muscles. By measuring each of the components of fitness before you start training and as you train you can measure your improvements—because standing on a scale is not going to tell you the condition of your heart, lungs, and muscles.

No matter what your current fitness level, goals, or interests, you have a lot of choices—and no excuses—when it comes to cardio/aerobic training: power walking, indoor cycling, outdoor cycling, using an elliptical machine, jogging, stair climbing, hiking, roller-skating, in-line skating, ice-skating, swimming, doing step class, taking dance class, kickboxing, doing interval/circuit training with weights, basketball, hockey, tennis, squash, racquetball, cross-country skiing, alpine skiing, snowboarding, soccer, and football. Choose the forms of cardio exercise that you enjoy so that you can stay active and healthy for life.

There are different levels of intensity you can aim for in your cardio/aerobic workout that will produce different results for your body. For our purposes, we're going to cover three key kinds of cardio/aerobic training, categorized by their intensity: aerobic base training, intermediate/advanced aerobic training, and interval training. (Remember the heart rate training zones you recorded in your Personal Fitness Profile? Here they are again!) The purpose of determining your own individual heart rate training zones is so you can train at the appropriate intensity to achieve your goals.

Regular cardiorespiratory/aerobic exercise provides virtually unlimited health benefits, including:

- improved heart and lung strength and function.
- higher overall energy and stamina.
- increased ability to use oxygen, which helps you burn fat.
- decreased levels of bad LDL cholesterol.
- enhanced sleep quality.
- a more-efficient metabolism.
- production of endorphins—"happy hormones," which are a hundred times better than any medication prescribed for depression or anxiety.
- elimination of toxins in the form of sweat.

AEROBIC/ANAEROBIC

The term *aerobic* literally means "with oxygen," and refers to the use of oxygen in muscles' energy-generating process. Aerobic exercise includes any type of exercise, typically performed at moderate levels of intensity for extended periods of time, that maintains an increased heart rate.

Anaerobic means "without oxygen." Anaerobic exercise is brief, high-intensity activity in which energy is being created without the use of oxygen; the by-products are lactic acid and hydrogen protons, which cause a burning sensation in the muscles being worked.

AEROBIC BASE TRAINING

Aerobic base is the heart-rate range where you can exercise comfortably for long periods of time (20 to 60 minutes or more) without stopping. This is the most important type of training for a beginning exerciser. Of the three types of training described here, this is the form that is lowest in intensity, requiring you to maintain a steady heart rate that is between 50 and 75 percent of your maximum heart rate for 20 minutes or longer. A half-hour power walk that elevates your heart rate to 65 percent of your maximum heart rate is a good example. During aerobic exercise, your body is using oxygen to create energy to keep going, oxygen that, in turn, your

MYTH: *I don't have time to get in 30 minutes of continuous cardio, so I am going to do 10 minutes at lunch, 10 minutes on my break, and 10 minutes at the end of the day.*

MYTH-BUSTER: Sorry, folks! You are just not going to get the same results as doing 30 minutes continuously. The effect on your muscles, heart, lungs, and hormonal system is completely different when you do your cardio exercise in one continuous session versus separating it into various parts of the day. Choosing to take a brief walk at lunch or climb the stairs is an added bonus of extra calories burned but it does not make up for your cardio session. Doing something is better than doing nothing, especially for beginners, but for best results, clear your mind, put on your workout clothes, grab your music, and put 110 percent into a full 30-minute cardio session. Pay yourself first!

body uses to burn fat and sugar. The more you condition your aerobic base, the more you will strengthen your heart and lungs, the more efficient you will become at using fat as a fuel source, and the easier it will be to function in your everyday life without running out of breath or energy. Just as you have to walk before you run, you have to train your aerobic base before you move up to higher intensities of training. You can use the calculation you made for your Aerobic Base Training Zone and program your heart-rate monitor with the upper and lower limits so you can keep track of your heart rate during your workout.

INTERMEDIATE-TO-ADVANCED AEROBIC TRAINING

As you progress with your workouts, you will see improvement in your heart and lung functions, oxygen consumption, and muscular endurance. After a while, working out in your Aerobic Base Training Zone will no longer challenge you. At this point, you need to up the intensity and elevate your heart rate to 65 to 85 percent of your maximum heart rate. As you increase intensity, make sure that you are always able to complete the exercises with good form and that you are feeling okay. You want to push yourself, but listen to your body: if you overexert, then you increase your risk of injury. If you ever feel light-headed or dizzy, then you should slow down your pace and lower your heart rate. Training at this intensity is a combination of aerobic and anaerobic, which means your body will create energy with and without oxygen. You will be burning fat and sugar as a fuel source, and you will be burning more calories per minute than in the aerobic base training. You will produce some lactic acid and hydrogen protons, which will create a burning sensation in your muscles but not enough to shut you down.

INTERVAL TRAINING

Interval training—high-intensity exercises, such as sprints, fast jogging, calisthenics, or heavier weights performed in short intervals of 15 seconds to 3 minutes—is a great way to keep your workouts compact, varied, complete, and energizing. As well as saving you time, working out in this way at a level of intensity of 70 to 90 percent of your maximum heart rate continues to rev your metabolism even after your workout is complete. This is the effect known as after burn, or excess postexercise oxygen consumption (EPOC). Once you reach a point where you can handle this kind of intensity, interval training is a great way to burn a lot of calories, change your physique, and keep your workouts exciting and your fitness level advancing.

. . .

Using various training intensities is one way we can make sure that we are overloading the body appropriately to create a physical change. Most exercise programs have only one intensity level, which will limit the amount your body can change. The Hollywood Trainer Weight-Loss Plan's exercise program has several levels because I don't want you to stop seeing results. The Cardio Burn workout has twelve levels; the Chest, Tri's, and Booty Circuit, five; the Back, Bi's, and Thighs Circuit, five; and the Core Workout, three. When your body starts to get used to the exercises, I want you to be able to take it to the next level and keep changing your body.

MUSCULAR STRENGTH AND MUSCULAR ENDURANCE

Muscular strength is the ability to exert maximum force, usually in a single repetition, or to execute strong or explosive movements like lifting a box, luggage, or children; catching yourself if you slip or fall; or pushing or pulling your body from a place of danger to one of safety when in an accident. People who are lacking in muscular strength will often injure themselves when trying to execute any of the above-mentioned movements because their muscles are too weak and deconditioned.

Muscular endurance is the ability to do several repetitions of a movement or to hold a particular position for an extended amount of time without injuring yourself or becoming fatigued. Muscular endurance is required every day to do basic functions for long periods of time like sitting upright at your desk, walking, and standing up with good posture. If you are weak in

---

MYTH: *I am going to lift only 3-pound weights because I don't want to get big.*

MYTH-BUSTER: Lifting 3-pound weights for all of your exercises is not going to put enough load on your body to create a change. It is imperative that you challenge your muscles by increasing the weight to 5, 8, or 10 pounds, or more. The weight should be heavy enough that by the time you complete the proper number of repetitions you can barely do two or three more. If you can repeat the exercise for five more repetitions, then the weight you are using is too light and it is time to increase the weight.

muscular endurance, you will often compensate with other muscle groups and create chronic injuries.

It is possible for someone to be conditioned in just one of the components discussed in this chapter. For example, an avid female weight-training participant has great muscular strength, so she can squat 150 pounds but she cannot jog for 3 miles because she has not trained her muscular endurance. A male marathon runner has great muscular endurance, so he can run 3 miles but he cannot squat 150 pounds because he has not trained his muscular strength.

Strength training, resistance training, or weight-lifting are the traditional methods used to improve muscular strength and muscular endurance. Muscular strength, which is the ability to exert maximum force, can also be trained through such activities as yoga, circuit training, sport-specific drills, plyometrics, and sprinting. Muscular endurance can be trained through Pilates, yoga, aqua aerobics, circuit training, kickboxing drills, sport-specific drills, dance technique drills, power walking, jogging, swimming, and hiking.

Many people don't include resistance training with weights in their workout regimen because they think it will bulk them up or that it won't help them lose weight. They are so *wrong*! It's actually extremely difficult to increase muscle mass, and your genetics play a major role; if it were easy there would be no billion-dollar industry in nutritional supplements, testosterone supplementation, human growth hormones, steroids, and super-protein products. Each of us is born with a finite number of muscle fibers that doesn't change throughout our lifetime. So while there are extreme resistance-training and nutritional measures one can take to significantly bulk up one's musculature, the kinds of resistance training you will be doing in my program will not give you Popeye arms or a bodybuilder's physique.

There are many reasons I advocate integrating resistance (or strength) training that effectively improves your muscular strength and muscular endurance, but the key three are:

1. Resistance training will help you *burn more body fat*. As you may recall from the section on proteins, the muscle cell is the site in the body where your body fat is burned off as fuel. The more actively you train and develop your muscles, the more fuel they will need. The more fuel they need, the more fat and sugar they will draw from the stores in your body, leaving less to settle in around your waistline! Strength training thus boosts your metabolism, helping you burn more calories even when you are at rest.

2. Strength training is important to *avoid injury and reduce stress on the body*. It is essential for your long-term, overall health to fortify the muscles, bones, and connective tissues

that form the infrastructure of your body. Every great athlete knows the importance of training their bodies so they are resilient enough to endure the stresses of their sport. *Your* body needs the same kind of preventive care. Whether you power walk, jog, cycle, step, hike, or simply run around with the kids, any cardio exercise that you are doing will put repetitive stress on your joints and bones—particularly your knees, ankles, and feet—and your lower back. The more weight you carry, the more stress you are putting on your body. If you take care to strengthen your body's framework, you will reduce your susceptibility to injury, as well as to serious problems like osteoporosis and arthritis.

3. Last but certainly not least, resistance training is the only way you're going to get that *beautiful, sexy, toned look*. By adding tension to your muscles, you can achieve the sculpted lines in your legs, butt, abs, and arms that you *know* you want. To make sure you achieve those beautiful sculpted lines, total body resistance training (muscular strength *and* muscular endurance) with dumbbells and calisthenics is integrated into the Chest, Tri's, and Booty Circuit; Back, Bi's, and Thighs Circuit; and Core Workout. It's time to get the body you want and deserve!

FLEXIBILITY

Flexibility is the most overlooked component of fitness, and the lack of it can cause common ailments like lower back pain, sciatica, shoulder impingement, and neck and shoulder stiffness. Your muscles contract (shorten) over and over again as you move through your daily activities. Many people suffer from overuse injuries caused by repeating the same movements for hours every day: sitting at a desk, typing at a computer, driving a car, carrying a baby, or even talking on the phone. A physical therapist will often treat repetitive-use injuries (and the muscle contractions that underlie them) with stretching exercises.

Stretching also helps relieve the muscle aches and pains caused by carrying excess weight, so it is critically important that you follow the Stretch-It-Out exercises outlined in Chapter 23 if you are just beginning on your weight-loss journey.

> Calisthenics are exercises that use the weight of your body
> for resistance, such as push-ups, lunges, and crunches.

Flexibility training also provides antiaging benefits. As you age, your muscles tighten, and your range of motion in a joint can be minimized. This can put a halt to active lifestyles and even hinder day-to-day activities.

And, finally, most people often overlook the aesthetic benefits of flexibility training—stretching will help you elongate your muscles so they do not have a bulky, bodybuilder look but a nice long, lean look, like a dancer's.

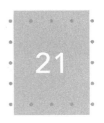

21

THE HOLLYWOOD TRAINER™ WEIGHT-LOSS PLAN EXERCISE PROGRAM

GETTING READY

Besides your own desire to make a change in your life and the information that you'll be getting from this book, there isn't much you're going to need to get started on my program. But before we plunge into the details, set yourself up for success with the following:

EQUIPMENT

The Hollywood Trainer Weight-Loss Plan's exercise program requires absolutely no fancy machinery or an expensive gym membership. You need only:

- an exercise mat
- a set of dumbbells that include 3-, 5-, 8-, 10-, 12-, and 15-pound weights. (You probably won't need anything higher than 15 pounds until you've been on my program for a while.)

You don't need to run out and buy any of those expensive exercise accessories that are on the market either: no step blocks, workout balls, or other fitness toys are necessary. My workouts are about getting back to basics and learning how to recruit your muscle fibers by improving your body awareness through proper form and technique. You will improve your cardiorespiratory health, muscular strength, muscular endurance—and flexibility. And if in the future you want to incorporate different fitness toys and equipment you will have established a solid foundation. You have to walk before you run.

WHAT TO WEAR

Wearing the right clothing will always help you enjoy and get the most out of your workout. You don't have to spend hundreds of dollars on fancy outfits, but you'll need to pick up a few pieces that are comfortable, fit you well, and help you feel confident. The best and longest-lasting clothes are made with Dri-Fit fabrics that pull your perspiration away from your skin so you don't feel damp. Many different companies have various names for Dri-Fit material, so it is important that you read the tags, which will describe the benefits of the material and clearly state whether the fabric has Dri-Fit qualities. And, if you want your workout gear to last, do not put it in the dryer—hang it to dry. (I have some Dri-Fit pieces that have lasted almost three years—and I work out almost every day.)

PROPER FOOTWEAR AND CARE

Equally important, if not more so, is what you wear on your feet. If you've been to a sports-supply store recently, you'll know what I mean when I say there's quite a selection of shoes to choose from. Your primary concern is whether or not the shoe is comfortable. If it's not comfortable when you are walking in the store, it is not going to suddenly become comfortable when you get home. It helps to figure out what kind of walking/running gait you have, since the way we walk or run puts stress on different parts of our feet, ankles, hips, and back. If you tend to walk with most of your weight on the outer edges of your feet, your feet will turn out slightly at the ankles—this is called supination, or underpronation. If you find that you walk with most of your weight centered at the inner edges of your feet, your feet will turn in slightly at the ankles—this is called pronation—or overpronation when the turn-in is extreme. To find out what your gait may have done to your body, take a pair of old sneakers that you've worn a lot, and put them together on a table. Looking at them from eye level, check to see if the shoes bend in or out noticeably. If your shoes have an outward tilt, you are an underpronator, whereas if your shoes have an inward tilt, you are a pronator or overpronator, depending on the tilt. If your shoes do not bend one way or the other, you have a neutral running gait. You can ask to have your gait examined at most running-shoe stores, which will help you get just the right shoe for your foot.

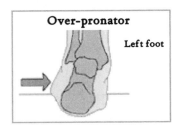

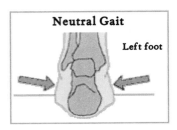

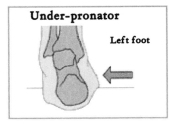

| If the shoes have a slight or significant inward tilt, then you exhibit an overpronation running gait. | If the shoes appear to be neutral and do not tilt inward or out, then you exhibit a neutral or normal running gait. | If the shoes have a slight or significant outward tilt, then you exhibit an underpronation (supination) running gait. |

Another common foot disorder is arch pain due either to flat feet or plantar fasciitis. If your entire foot comes into near-complete contact with the ground every time you take a step, you should use flat-foot insoles and orthotics to help you alleviate discomfort. Plantar fasciitis is a repetitive stress disorder that results in an inflammation of the connective tissue and muscles in the sole of the foot. People who are overweight are especially susceptible to plantar fasciitis. Insoles and orthotics are available to correct the problem. You should never work out on painful feet. Not only will your whole form be out of whack, but you are also more vulnerable to injury. Remember, you have only one pair of feet, and they do a lot for you, so take care of them.

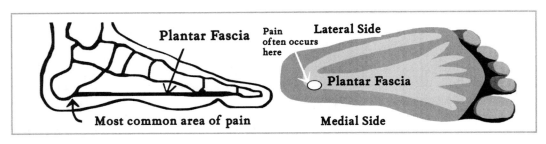

Plantar Fasciitis

By now you have heard a lot about the positive aspects of this program and several of the elements that have been included to maximize your results. Now it's time to provide you with the exercise program set out in a weekly plan of various exercises. The Hollywood Trainer Weight-Loss Plan Exercise Program is a seven-day plan that includes five different workouts specifically designed to help you lose weight, and sculpt, define, and tone your muscles, with an extra emphasis on the abdominals.

This program will produce results for you now, and for months and even years into the future. In Part 3: 21 Days That Will Change Your Life, on each day you are required to execute a specific workout as outlined above. You will have to come to this section to follow the photos and exercise descriptions for the specific daily workouts. Each of the five workouts that make up the program—Cardio Burn; Stretch-It-Out; Chest, Tri's, and Booty (Circuit A); Core; and Back, Bi's, and Thighs (Circuit B)—is described in the following chapters with photos and written descriptions to show you how to execute each exercise effectively, with good form and technique. (All the exercises are also shown on *The Hollywood Trainer Weight-Loss Plan Workout* DVD.)

THIS IS THE HOLLYWOOD TRAINER WEIGHT-LOSS PLAN'S EXERCISE PROGRAM

Day 1: Cardio Burn; Stretch-It-Out

Day 2: Chest, Tri's, and Booty (Circuit A); Core; Stretch-It-Out

Day 3: Cardio Burn; Stretch-It-Out

Day 4: Back, Bi's, and Thighs (Circuit B); Core; Stretch-It-Out

Day 5: Chest, Tri's, and Booty (Circuit A); Stretch-It-Out

Day 6: Back, Bi's, and Thighs (Circuit B); Core; Stretch-It-Out

Day 7: Rest, Relax, and Rejuvenate

This illustration, which shows the major muscle groups in your body, will help you learn the names of each muscle so you will know which one I refer to in the exercises.

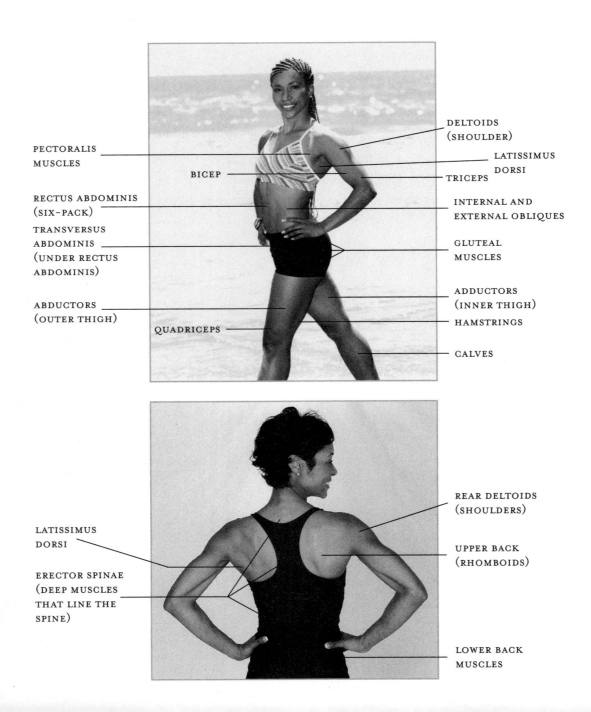

22

CARDIO BURN

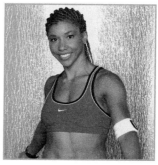

This Cardio Burn workout has twelve levels designed to burn calories, burn fat, tone your abs and legs, and improve your aerobic base. Level 1 starts with a basic 20-minute power walk, so there's no need to be intimidated, and Level 12 incorporates intervals of jogging and sprinting or power walking on an incline, so no matter what level of cardiorespiratory fitness you are at, I have the right level for you. I recommend that everyone start at Level 1 unless you have been exercising on a regular basis, in which case you can look at the description of each level and choose the level that best reflects your current cardio regimen.

From Levels 2 to 12 I have provided you with both high-impact and low-impact options. The high-impact exercise is a combination of walking and jogging or jogging and sprinting, the low-impact a combination of walking flat and walking on an incline. It is important to listen to your body. Some days you may feel pain in your ankles or knees, or you may be suffering from an injury and your doctor has specifically stated that you should not run or jump. You can still get a great workout doing the low-impact activity of walking on an incline without putting excessive stress on your joints compared to jogging or sprinting. Choose the option that is best for your body. If you are carrying a lot of excess weight then I highly recommend choosing the low-impact options of walking and walking on an incline. As soon as you drop some weight and strengthen your joints you can slowly progress to the high-impact options.

Pull the Cardiorespiratory Training Log (Form 8) from your personal journal (Form 8 can be photocopied from the Appendix or you can download it at www.thehollywoodtrainer.com) and review the points in the workout where you are required to track your heart rate. You need to track your heart rate to monitor your level of intensity. Refer to your heart-rate training zones as recorded in your Personal Fitness Profile (Form 6) and make sure you transfer your individual heart-rate training zones onto your Cardiorespiratory Training Log. Tracking your heart rate each time you do the Cardio Burn workout will help you learn more about your body, your heart, and your level of fitness. As soon as your heart rate remains between 50 percent and 60 percent of your maximum heart rate for the entire workout, or you feel like you are not being challenged, then it is time to take it to the next level. Remember the principles of exercise training at the beginning of this part of the book: if you don't challenge yourself then you will not see results!

THE 7-DAY HOLLYWOOD TRAINER WEIGHT-LOSS PLAN WORKOUT

Day 1: **Cardio-Burn;** Stretch-It-Out

Day 2: Chest, Tri's, and Booty (Circuit A); Core; Stretch-It-Out

Day 3: **Cardio Burn;** Stretch-It-Out

Day 4: Back, Bi's, and Thighs (Circuit B); Core; Stretch-It-Out

Day 5: Chest, Tri's, and Booty (Circuit A); Stretch-It-Out

Day 6: Back, Bi's, and Thighs (Circuit B); Core; Stretch-It-Out

Day 7: Rest, Relax, and Rejuvenate

WARM-UP

Each level begins with a 3- to 5-minute warm-up and stretches. A warm-up consists of walking at a slow to moderate pace to just get the blood circulating to the muscles and get the body warm and ready for a more vigorous workout. As soon as your body is warm move into the following stretches: straddle stretch, hamstring stretch, quadriceps stretch, cross-legged stretch, buttocks stretch, lower-back cat stretch, and calf stretch. All of these stretches are outlined in the Stretch-It-Out section with photos and descriptions. Hold each stretch for only 8 to 10 seconds because we don't want your body to cool down. All of these stretches should take you about 2 minutes to complete. The purpose of the warm-up and stretches is to decrease your risk of injury as you move into more-vigorous exercise.

COOLDOWN

Once you complete the vigorous part of the workout it is necessary to do a 3- to 5-minute cooldown. For the cooldown you need to slow down your pace so that your heart rate can return to below 50 percent of your max heart rate. The cooldown will help your blood move from your extremities back to the core of your body so you do not experience blood pooling. Blood pooling in your legs or arms causes cramping and may occur if you stop exercising abruptly without a cooldown. The cooldown will also increase oxygen to your muscles to help get rid of lactic acid, and prevent dizziness and nausea.

Once you have cooled down, stretch your muscles by following all of the exercises in the Stretch-It-Out workout. Hold each stretch for 1 to 30 seconds to help decrease stiffness and muscle soreness. The cooldown and stretches are also very important to help you take a moment of peace to reflect on the accomplishment of the workout you just completed and prepare your mind and spirit to enter another day with a positive attitude.

MYTH: *I need to be sweating a lot to know that I am working hard and losing weight.*

MYTH-BUSTER: Sweating is your body's cooling mechanism, and it just means that you are really hot and your body needs to cool off. The weight you lose from sweating is just water weight. You can drop as much as five to ten pounds of water weight if you are exercising in very hot or extremely hot conditions. Excess heat and water loss leave you feeling tired and sluggish and at risk for heat exhaustion or heat stroke. Water is needed to burn fat, so if you are exercising in very hot conditions make sure you hydrate yourself and replenish your body. Don't be fooled. You are not burning extra fat, you are just losing precious water.

CARDIO BURN WORKOUT

The Cardio Burn Workout is done on Day 1 and Day 3.

LEVEL	WARM-UP	EXERCISE(S)	COOLDOWN
1	3- to 5-minute power walk	20–minute power walk	3–5 minutes
2	3- to 5-minute power walk	3-minute power walk; 60- to 90-second jog or treadmill incline to 6.0; repeat 6 times	3–5 minutes
3	3- to 5-minute power walk	2-minute power walk; 2-minute jog or treadmill incline to 6.0; repeat 6 times	3–5 minutes
4	3- to 5-minute power walk	2-minute power walk; 3-minute jog or treadmill incline to 6.0; repeat 6 times	3–5 minutes
5	3- to 5-minute power walk	1-minute power walk; 3-minute jog or treadmill incline to 6.0; repeat 7 times	3–5 minutes
6	3- to 5-minute power walk	1-minute power walk; 5-minute jog or treadmill incline to 6.0; repeat 4 times	3–5 minutes
7	3- to 5-minute power walk	2-minute power walk; 15-minute jog or treadmill incline to 6.0; repeat 2 times	3–5 minutes
8	3- to 5-minute power walk	30-minute jog or treadmill incline to 6.0	3–5 minutes
9	3- to 5-minute power walk	5-minute jog or treadmill incline to 6.0; 60-second run/sprint or treadmill incline to 10.0; repeat 4 times	3–5 minutes
10	3- to 5-minute power walk	5-minute jog or treadmill incline to 6.0; 90-second run/sprint or treadmill incline to 10.0; repeat 4 times	3–5 minutes
11	3- to 5-minute power walk	5-minute jog or treadmill incline to 6.0; 2-minute run/sprint or treadmill incline to 10.0; repeat 4 times	3–5 minutes
12	3- to 5-minute power walk	5-minute jog or treadmill incline to 6.0; 2-minute run/sprint or treadmill incline to 10.0; repeat 5 times	3–5 minutes

23

STRETCH-IT-OUT

The purpose of the Stretch-It-Out is to provide you with stretches that you can do during the warm-ups and cooldowns as well as a complete flexibility workout on its own that will help you improve your flexibility.

THE 7-DAY HOLLYWOOD TRAINER WEIGHT-LOSS PLAN WORKOUT

Day 1: Cardio Burn; **Stretch-It-Out**
Day 2: Chest, Tri's, and Booty (Circuit A); Core; **Stretch-It-Out**
Day 3: Cardio Burn; **Stretch-It-Out (Flexibility Stretching)**
Day 4: Back, Bi's, and Thighs (Circuit B); Core; **Stretch-It-Out**
Day 5: Chest, Tri's, and Booty (Circuit A); **Stretch-It-Out**
Day 6: Back, Bi's, and Thighs (Circuit B); Core; **Stretch-It-Out**
Day 7: Rest, Relax, and Rejuvenate

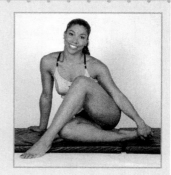

WARM-UP STRETCHING

After you have completed a 3- to 5-minute warm-up as indicated in each of your workouts, do the designated stretches for that particular workout. Each workout is designed to work particular muscle groups, so it is important to stretch those muscles after they have been warmed up to decrease your risk of injury. For example, in the warm-up section of the Cardio Burn workout you are required to do specific stretches for the muscles in your lower back and legs, holding each for a shorter period than in the full Stretch-It-Out workout.

COOLDOWN STRETCHING

After you have completed a 3- to 5-minute cooldown, do all of the stretches in the Stretch-It-Out workout. Hold each stretch for 15 to 30 seconds. The purpose of the cooldown stretches is to help decrease muscle soreness and stiffness. Stretching after the workout also gives you an opportunity to have a few moments of peace. At the end of your workout your body will be loaded with happy hormones (endorphins) and you'll be feeling great. It is important that you take advantage of the happy-hormone high to help motivate you through the day, which is another reason I recommend starting your day with a workout. During the stretching, you can achieve a spiritually relaxing frame of mind; recognize your accomplishments of completing your workout; give thanks for another day with good health; clear any negative thoughts; and prepare yourself to have an amazing positive day.

MYTH: *Stretching isn't going to help me get smaller, so I can skip the stretches.*

MYTH-BUSTER: Stretching will help you elongate your muscles so they do not have a bulky, bodybuilder look but a nice long, lean look, like a dancer's. Stretching will also help relieve some of your aches and pains from carrying excess weight, from regular daily activities, and from excess stress and strain on your muscles.

FLEXIBILITY STRETCHING

To improve your flexibility it is necessary to hold your stretches for a longer period of time than 8 to 10 seconds or 15 to 30 seconds. To lengthen your muscle fibers you have to overload them just as you do when you are strengthening them. Remember the Overload principle? It applies here just as it does in the more rigorous workouts. You will never observe a dancer or yoga student hold a stretch for only 8 to 10 seconds, because they know that in order to improve their flexibility it is necessary to hold or work a stretch or pose for an extended period of time of at least 1 to 3 minutes to really tear down those muscle fibers and get them to lengthen. Holding stretches for 1 to 3 minutes can create muscle soreness just like lifting weights or jogging. You are putting an excess stress or load onto your body and it is making a physiological adaptation.

Just as there are different levels of intensity for cardio exercise, there are also levels of intensity for stretching. If you hold a stretch for too long and you have never held stretches before, you can actually cause muscle soreness and muscle stiffness. It is important to gradually progress in the length of time that you hold a stretch. Start with holding each stretch for 30 to 45 seconds and then measure how your body feels the next day. If you feel fine, then the next time you do the flexibility stretching hold each stretch for 45 to 60 seconds and continue to progress until you finally reach 3 to 5 minutes. Remember that this is the prescription for flexibility stretching to lengthen your muscle fibers, which is different from the brief stretches that you will do in the warm-ups and cooldowns. (The Stretch-It-Out workout provided on *The Hollywood Trainer Weight-Loss Plan* DVD is executed in this format, which makes it a 40-minute flexibility workout.)

The Stretch-It-Out workout is done on Days 1 through 6. However, on Day 3 you are required to hold the stretches for 1 to 3 minutes (Flexibility Stretching) at the end of the Cardio Burn workout. On all of the other days you are just required to do the Stretch-It-Out exercises holding for 8 to 10 seconds and/or as part of the warm-up and cooldown as indicated in each workout.

THE BREATH

The breath is extremely important for all exercise, but it is even more significant in stretching. Taking deep steady breaths will help you:

- Bring oxygen into the body so you can flush out toxins that are in the bloodstream, muscles, and joints.
- Release tension so you can lengthen your muscles.
- Allow you to focus your energy so you can enjoy the meditative, relaxing benefits of stretching.

  Proper breathing is necessary to help you maximize the results of the stretches. Your breathing should be deep and steady, with each inhale and exhale lasting 4 to 5 seconds. During each inhale/exhale cycle you should focus on the muscles that you are stretching. I recommend that beginners start with 3 to 4 breaths (inhale/exhale cycle) or 30 to 45 seconds for each stretch and then progress to an average cycle of 5 to 8 breaths or 45 to 60 seconds per stretch. If you have a specific area that needs extra lengthening, you can progress to hold those stretches for 15 to 20 breaths or 3 to 5 minutes.

THE STRETCHES

• STRADDLE STRETCH

Sit tall on the floor with your legs open as wide as you can without bending the knees and feet flexed (not pointed). Inhale as you pull in your abdominals and lean forward toward the floor, leading with the chest (i.e., don't round your back) and place your hands on the floor. (Imagine there is a string pulling the crown of your head, which is pulling your neck and spine into a nice long line.) Hold that position for at least 3 deep inhales and exhales. On each exhale try to reach your fingers a little bit farther so you feel a deeper stretch in the inner thighs and hamstrings. Do not round your back: keep your spine long and the abdominals tight.

Return to the starting position, sitting tall with your shoulders stacked over your hips.

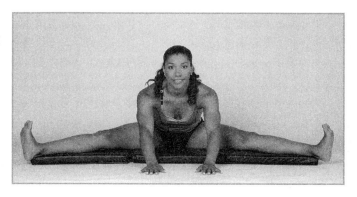

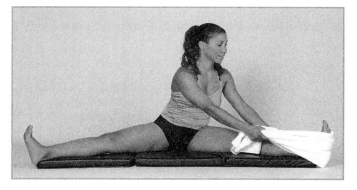

Inhale and pull your abdominals tight as you lengthen your spine. Exhale as you rotate your shoulders so they are square to your right foot. Inhale and reach your arms up overhead. Exhale as you reach forward toward your right foot, bending at your hips. (You do not need to touch your foot if you cannot do so easily.) Inhale as you hold the stretch, then exhale and try to reach a little bit farther without rounding your back as you feel the stretch in your inner thighs, lower back, hips, and hamstrings. Continue to hold the stretch for 3 to 4 more breaths, pushing the stretch a little farther with each exhalation. To help you hold the stretch, hold a towel or stretching strap with both hands and wrap it around the ball of your foot. The idea is not to put your head on your knee but to feel the stretch that is best for your body. Repeat the stretch sequence on the other leg.

• FORWARD FLEXION HAMSTRING STRETCH (WITH ONE KNEE BENT)

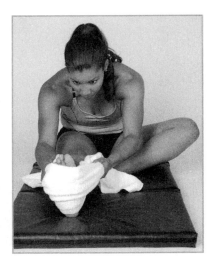

Sit on your buttocks (sitz bones) and extend your right leg straight in front of you. Bend your left knee and rest the bottom of your left foot against the inside of your knee or inner thigh.

Inhale and reach your arms up overhead, lengthening your spine and pulling in your abdominals. Exhale as you reach your arms forward, without rounding your back, as far as you can and then hold that position. Inhale and hold the stretch; exhale as you try to reach a little bit farther as you feel a stretch in your right hamstring, left hip, and lower back. Continue to hold the stretch for 3 to 4 more deep breaths. To help you maintain the stretch, hold a towel or stretching strap with both hands and wrap it around the ball of your foot. Repeat the stretch on the other leg.

• SIDE LYING QUADRICEPS STRETCH

Lie down on your left side, resting your head on your left arm. Your body should be in a straight line from head to toe.

Bend your right leg behind you and grasp your right foot with your right hand, pulling your right foot toward your buttocks and holding it to create a stretch in your right quadriceps (front of your thigh). Inhale as you pull your abdominals in and lengthen your spine; exhale as you hold the stretch. Continue to breathe for 3 to 4 more cycles. Repeat the stretch on the other leg.

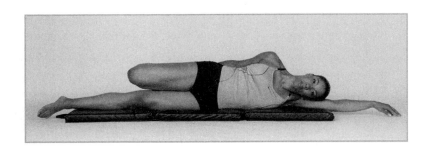

OUTER THIGH CROSS-LEGGED STRETCH

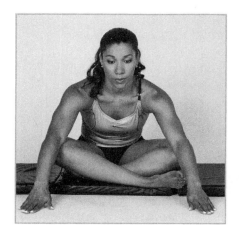 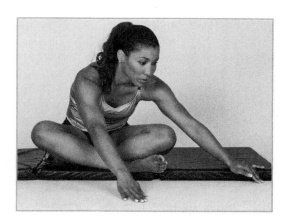

Sit on the floor in a comfortable cross-legged position with your right leg crossed in front of your left, back straight, and abs tight. Inhale. Relax your neck and shoulders. Exhale as you reach your arms forward until you feel a stretch in your hips. Hold this stretch for 3 to 4 full breaths.

Return to the starting position, then reach both arms to your left side in front of your left knee without lifting your right buttock off the floor. You should feel a deeper stretch in your right hip. Hold this position and continue to breathe 3 to 4 cycles. On each exhale, try to reach farther away from your body, but keep your back as straight as you can. Repeat the same stretch sequence with the left leg in front, focusing the stretch on the left hip.

• HAMSTRING STRETCH (LYING ON BACK)

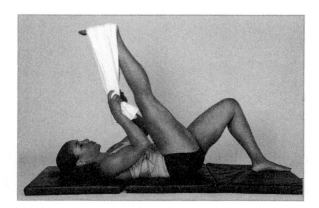

Lie on your back with your knees bent, feet on the floor close to your buttocks. With bent knee, lift your right leg off the ground and wrap a towel or stretching strap around the bottom of your right foot. Inhale, keeping your neck and shoulders on the floor and relaxed. Exhale as you extend your right leg straight up in the air, holding on to the ends of the towel or stretching strap. Continue to inhale and exhale and try to deepen the stretch by pulling the right leg closer to your body. Continue to hold the stretch for 3 to 4 more breaths. Repeat the stretch with the other leg.

• BUTTOCKS STRETCH (LYING ON BACK)

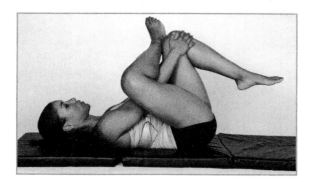

Lie on your back with your knees bent, both feet on the floor close to your buttocks. Place your right ankle on your left thigh just above the knee, externally rotating your right hip. Inhale, keeping your neck and shoulders relaxed and on the floor. Grasp the left leg on the hamstrings just above the knee with both hands, exhale, and lift your left foot off the ground, bringing your legs closer to your chest. You should feel a comfortable stretch in your right buttocks and outer hip area (gluteus medius, gluteus maximus, external hip rotators, iliotibial band, abductors, and lower back). Hold this stretch for 3 to 4 deep breaths. Repeat the stretch on the other leg.

◦ SPINAL ROTATION STRETCH (LYING ON THE BACK)

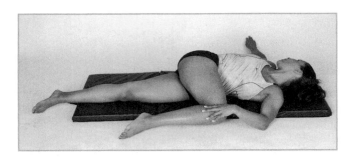

Lie on your back, legs straight and together, arms at your side. Inhale and relax. On your first exhale, bring your right knee into your chest, stretching your hamstring and lower back. Hold your knee in this position by placing both hands on top of your right shin. Continue to hold this position for 3 to 4 full breaths. Keeping your right leg bent, on your next exhale rotate your torso to the left until your right knee touches (or is close to touching) the ground on your left side. Try to keep your right shoulder on the ground for the deepest stretch, but listen to your body and rotate only as far as needed to feel a nice stretch in your lower back. Hold for 3 to 4 deep breaths, trying to go a little deeper with each exhale. Return to the starting position and repeat the stretch on the other side by pulling the left knee into your chest and rotating to your right.

COBRA (ABDOMINAL) STRETCH

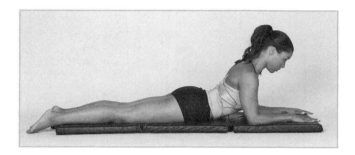

Lie facedown, forehead touching the floor. Place your palms next to your shoulders with your elbows resting close to your torso. Inhale and lengthen your body into a nice long line by pointing your toes, extending—but not lifting—your legs and lengthening your neck. (Imagine there is a string attached to the crown of your head and it is pulling your spine in a straight line like the shape of a torpedo.) Inhale and exhale two more times holding this lengthened position. On your next exhale, gently push through the palms of your hands, lifting your chest off the floor. Lift as high as you can without feeling any strain or pain in your lower back. In this Cobra stretch position you should feel a stretch through your abdominals (rectus abdominis). Continue to hold the stretch for 3 to 4 more breaths. Roll down to the start position. Repeat this total stretch sequence one more time.

CAT (LOWER BACK) STRETCH

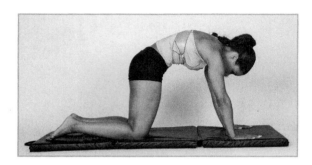

Come to your hands and knees to create a box shape. Inhale, pulling your navel to your spine, and lengthen your neck and your spine into a straight line parallel to the floor. Exhale and continue to contract your abdominals as you round your spine as high as you can toward the ceiling, allowing your head to drop toward your chest—like the shape of a stretching cat. Inhale as you return to the starting position, releasing the stretch and making the spine parallel to the floor. Exhale and round the spine, inhale and lengthen the spine. Repeat the sequence 3 to 4 more times.

SEATED CALF STRETCH

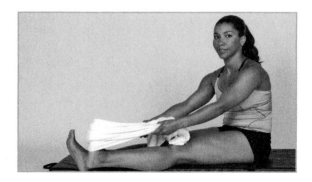

Sit tall on the floor with your legs spread comfortably apart and feet flexed (dorsiflexion). Hook your towel or stretching strap around the ball of your left foot. Keep your back as straight as you can as you exhale, and apply additional pressure by pulling the towel toward you until you feel a good stretch in your calf and Achilles tendon. Hold the stretch and continue to breathe for 3 to 4 breaths. Repeat the stretch on the other calf.

• CHEST AND FRONT DELTOID STRETCH

Sitting on your buttocks (or standing), roll your shoulders back and down and interlace your fingers behind your back. Inhale and relax your neck; exhale as you lift your arms up and away from your back, opening and stretching your chest (pectoralis minor and major) and front shoulder muscles (anterior deltoids). Hold the stretch for 3 to 4 breaths.

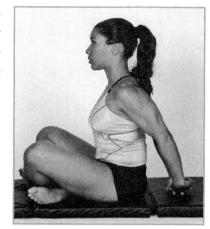

• BICEP AND FOREARM STRETCH

Standing or sitting tall, extend your left arm straight out in front of you with forearm and palm facing up. Gently apply pressure to the fingertips of your left hand with your right hand until you feel a stretch in your left forearm and left bicep. Hold the stretch for 3 to 4 breaths, then repeat the stretch on the other arm.

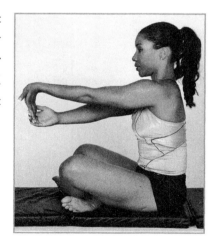

TRICEPS STRETCH

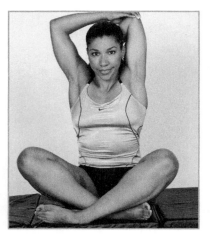

Standing or sitting tall, raise your right arm above your head, bend at the elbow, and place your right palm on your upper back between your shoulder blades as if you were going to give yourself a pat on the back. With your left hand apply pressure to the top of your right elbow until you feel a stretch in the back of your right arm (triceps). As you hold the stretch, keep your spine and neck long and straight, pressing your head gently but firmly into your right arm. Be careful not to drop your posture. Hold the stretch for 3 to 4 breaths, then repeat on the other arm.

UPPER BACK STRETCH

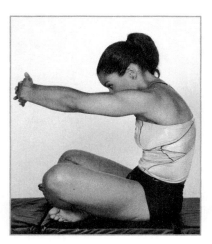

Standing or sitting tall, imagine you are wrapping your arms around an extra-large beach ball at chest height and interlace your fingers. Inhale and pull your navel to your spine; exhale as you round your spine and contract your abs, pressing energy away from your body through your arms until you feel a nice stretch in your upper back. Repeat this movement for 3 to 4 more breaths. For a deeper upper back stretch you can also try this same movement holding on to a fixed object like a stair rail, light pole, gym machine, or fence.

REAR DELTOID AND TRICEPS STRETCH

Standing or sitting tall, cross your left arm in front of your chest with your forearm and palm facing toward you. Place your right hand against your left upper arm just above your elbow. Gently apply pressure to your left arm, keeping it close to your body, until you feel a stretch in your left shoulder (rear deltoid) and triceps. Remember to relax your neck and press your shoulders down away from your neck. Hold this stretch for 3 to 4 more breaths, then repeat the stretch on the other arm.

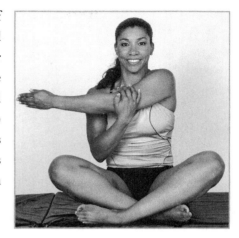

• NECK STRETCH SEQUENCE 1-2-3

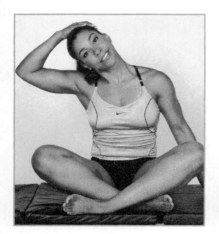 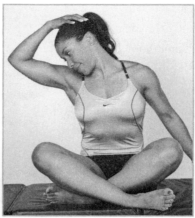 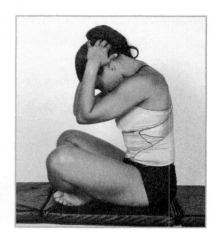

Standing or sitting up tall, bend your right arm over your head until your right hand is resting against the left side of your head just above your left ear. Inhale and hold the position, lengthening your neck in an easy stretch; exhale as you drop your right ear toward your right shoulder and apply pressure gently to the left side of your head with your right hand as you feel a deeper stretch in the left side of your neck. Hold this position for 3 to 4 more breaths.

On the next exhale, gently roll your chin to the top of your right chest. Hold this position and feel a deeper stretch, involving different neck muscle fibers. Hold this position for 3 to 4 more breaths.

Keeping your chin on the right chest, move your hand to the middle of the back of your head and gently apply downward pressure until you feel a deeper stretch, working different neck muscle fibers. Hold this position for 3 to 4 breaths.

Interlace your fingers behind your head and drop your chin forward, gently applying pressure to the back of your head until you feel a stretch in the back of your neck. Hold this position for 3 to 4 breaths. Repeat the entire sequence on the other side.

24

CHEST, TRI'S, AND BOOTY
(CIRCUIT A)

THE 7-DAY HOLLYWOOD TRAINER
WEIGHT-LOSS PLAN WORKOUT

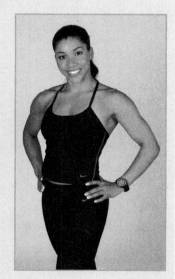

Day 1: Cardio Burn; Stretch-It-Out

Day 2: **Chest, Tri's, and Booty (Circuit A);** Core; Stretch-It-Out

Day 3: Cardio Burn; Stretch-It-Out (Flexibility Stretching)

Day 4: Back, Bi's, and Thighs (Circuit B); Core; Stretch-It-Out

Day 5: **Chest, Tri's, and Booty (Circuit A);** Stretch-It-Out

Day 6: Back, Bi's, and Thighs (Circuit B); Core; Stretch-It-Out

Day 7: Rest, Relax, and Rejuvenate

CIRCUIT TRAINING

The Chest, Tri's, and Booty (Circuit A) is designed to help you burn calories and fat to sculpt and define your chest, shoulders, triceps, buttocks, quadriceps, abdominals, and hamstrings. This workout, as well as the Back, Bi's, and Thighs (Circuit B), incorporates resistance training in a circuit-training format. Circuit training is proven to be one of the most effective methods of training for weight loss; it has you moving from one exercise to another in fast succession. Because your body is constantly moving, your heart rate remains elevated the entire time, which means that you will also be getting many of the benefits of a cardio workout. Most important, you will be burning more calories during and after your workout than you can do with resistance training alone. Circuit training also saves you time by allowing you to work one muscle group while another is recuperating. Finally, circuit training with several levels of intensity ensures that you will never plateau. The constant variety and progression keep your mind engaged and your body challenged, which only increases the calories you'll burn and the long-term benefits you'll reap. This particular workout has five levels. I recommend that you start at the first level and then progress to the next when you can complete all of the exercises with good form and technique, when you can complete all of the sets and repetitions required for that level, or when you feel like you are no longer being challenged.

MYTH: *I have to do cardio first to lose some weight, and then I will tone up with weights later.*

MYTH-BUSTER: You will burn more calories and have more of a physical change in your body if you incorporate cardio and resistance training at the beginning of your program.

As you complete each circuit series, fill in the required information in your Circuit Training Log (copy Form 9 in the Appendix or download it from www.thehollywoodtrainer.com). It is important to record the amount of weight you are using for each specific exercise, the number of repetitions you complete of each movement, and your heart rate at specific points of the workout. All of this information will help you see your progress and decide when it is time to take it to the next level.

Target muscles: chest, shoulders, triceps/butt, quads, abs, and hamstrings

Equipment: dumbbells (beginner: 3 to 5 pounds; intermediate: 5 to 8 pounds; advanced: 5 to 25 pounds), an exercise mat, and a chair (optional, to help you balance while doing the reverse lunges).

Warm-up and stretch: Start your workout with a 3- to 5-minute warm-up. Power walking, stationary bike, or cardio machine are optional warm-ups. Complete all of the stretches in the Stretch-It-Out workout, holding each for 8 to10 seconds. (*The Hollywood Trainer Weight-Loss Plan Workout* DVD has a 5-minute warm-up and stretch using total body aerobic movements that you can also use.)

Exercise Rx: Repeat each circuit twice (2 sets) and then immediately move on to the next circuit. Take a break between exercises and circuits only if you need to. If you complete the specified number of repetitions of an exercise and feel that you can still lift your weight at least 5 more times, you should increase the weight the next time you do the workout. (Remember the Overload principle.)

Cooldown: After you have completed your circuit workout, lower your heart rate by marching on the spot or taking a slow walk for 3 to 5 minutes. Repeat all of the stretches in the Stretch-It-Out workout, holding each stretch for 15 to 30 seconds. (*The Hollywood Trainer Weight-Loss Plan Workout* DVD has a 5-minute cooldown and stretch that you can also use.)

I recommend following *The Hollywood Trainer Weight-Loss Plan Workout* DVD to learn the correct form and technique of each of the exercises in the Chest, Tri's, and Booty (Circuit A). One set of each circuit is performed on the DVD, which is very well organized so you can complete the exercises for the level at which you are working and then repeat it from the top to complete two sets.

You are required to do Chest, Tri's, and Booty (Circuit A) on Day 2 and Day 5 of the weekly exercise program.

CHEST, TRI'S, AND BOOTY (CIRCUIT A) SERIES: LEVEL 1

Complete 2 sets of each circuit.

CIRCUIT 1	10–25 from-the-knee push-ups; 30-second plank
	15 back kicks on all fours
	15 basic crunches
CIRCUIT 2	15 chest flys
	15 reverse lunges (chair for balance)
	15 repeater knees
CIRCUIT 3	15 overhead presses
	15 squats; 30-second chair pose
	15 alternating knee-ups

MYTH: *All of my muscle has turned to fat.*

MYTH-BUSTER: Muscle and fat are two different tissues. When you are not exercising, your muscles decrease in size, and when you overeat, your excess calories are packed away into your fat (adipose) tissue.

CHEST, TRI'S, AND BOOTY (CIRCUIT A) SERIES: LEVEL 2

This level increases the reps and incorporates small changes to the exercises to make them more challenging. Get rid of the chair you used for balance in Level 1. Balance comes from your core; focus on pulling your navel to your spine and contracting your abdominals to help you balance.

Drop sets are also new in this level. Chest flys and overhead presses are performed in drop sets: do the first 15 reps with the heaviest weight you can lift with good form, and then immediately drop down to a lighter weight (25 to 50 percent less weight) to do 10 more reps. Drop sets help you achieve more tone and definition, because you are recruiting more muscle fiber types. The more muscle fiber types you engage, the more muscle teardown and muscle cell rejuvenation will occur and the more tension will be created in the muscle. As an added bonus, you also burn more calories.

Complete 2 sets of each circuit.

CIRCUIT 1	25 from-the-knee push-ups; 30-second plank 25 back kicks on all fours 25 basic crunches
CIRCUIT 2	Drop set chest flys: 15 reps max weight, drop weight 25–50% for 10 more reps 15 reverse lunges, no chair 25 repeater knees
CIRCUIT 3	Drop set overhead presses: 15 reps max weight, drop weight 25–50% for 10 more reps 25 squats; 30-second chair pose 25 alternating knee-ups

CHEST, TRI'S, AND BOOTY (CIRCUIT A) SERIES: LEVEL 3

Now it's time to increase reps again and modify some of the exercises to make them more challenging—no more from-the-knees push-ups, it's military style from here on out! It's also time to add a fourth circuit.

Complete 2 sets of each circuit.

CIRCUIT 1	10–15 push-ups; 30-second plank
	25 back kicks on all fours
	25 basic crunches
CIRCUIT 2	Drop set chest flys: 15 reps max weight, drop weight 25–50% for 10 more reps
	20 reverse lunges
	25 repeater knees
CIRCUIT 3	Drop set overhead presses: 15 reps max weight, drop weight 25–50% for 10 more reps
	25 squats; 60-second chair pose
	25 alternating knee-ups
CIRCUIT 4	15 overhead triceps extensions
	10 single leg reaches
	15 standing oblique crunches

CHEST, TRI'S, AND BOOTY (CIRCUIT A) SERIES: LEVEL 4

This level adds reps to some of the exercises, and one more circuit. Complete 2 sets of each circuit.

CIRCUIT 1	15 push-ups
	25 back kicks on all fours
	25 basic crunches
CIRCUIT 2	Drop set chest flys: 15 reps max weight, drop weight 25–50% for 10 more reps
	20 reverse lunges
	25 repeater knees
CIRCUIT 3	Drop set overhead presses: 15 reps max weight, drop weight 25–50% for 10 more reps
	25 squats; 60-second chair pose
	25 alternating knee-ups
CIRCUIT 4	Drop set overhead triceps extension: 15 reps max weight, drop weight 25–50% for 10 more reps
	15 single leg reaches
	25 standing oblique crunches
CIRCUIT 5	15 triceps kickbacks
	10 single leg squats
	15 cross-torso repeater knees

CHEST, TRI'S, AND BOOTY (CIRCUIT A) SERIES: LEVEL 5

Congratulations! You've achieved an advanced level of fitness. This level adds reps to the final circuit because you need to be challenged one more time. You should be feeling great.

Complete 2 sets of each circuit.

CIRCUIT 1	25 push-ups; 30-second plank 25 back kicks on all fours 25 basic crunches
CIRCUIT 2	Straight set 25 chest flys, or drop set chest flys: 15 reps max weight, drop weight 25–50% for 10 more reps 25 reverse lunges 25 repeater knees
CIRCUIT 3	Drop set overhead presses: 15 reps max weight, drop weight 25–50% for 10 more reps 25 squats; 60-second chair pose 25 alternating knee-ups
CIRCUIT 4	Straight set 25 triceps extensions, or drop set triceps extensions: 15 reps max weight, drop weight 25–50% for 10 more reps 15 single leg reaches 25 standing oblique crunches
CIRCUIT 5	Drop set triceps kickbacks: 15 reps max weight, drop weight 25–50% for 10 more reps 15 single leg squats 25 cross-torso repeater knees

CHEST, TRI'S, AND BOOTY (CIRCUIT A) EXERCISES

All of these exercises are demonstrated on *The Hollywood Trainer Weight-Loss Plan Workout* DVD. I recommend following the DVD at least once to help learn good form and technique. Just click to the chapter on the DVD that is labeled "Chest, Tri's, and Booty (Circuit A)" and you can follow along with your book because they are in the exact same order.

PUSH-UP (FROM KNEES OR TOES) AND PLANK

(Levels 1 to 5)

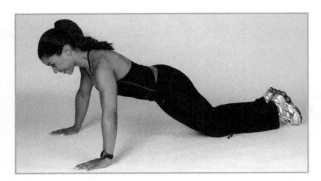
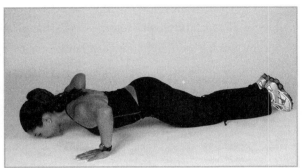
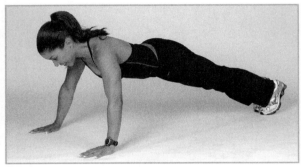
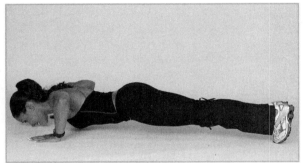

Place your knees on a mat and place hands slightly wider than shoulders. Extend spine long so there is a straight line from the crown of your head, through your spine, and through your legs to your knees (or your toes—full push-up—if you are able to hold this position). Always pull your abs in tight to help protect your back.

Keeping your spine long and torso straight and strong, inhale and lower your chest toward the floor by bending your elbows, resisting your body weight using the muscles in your chest, shoulders, biceps, and triceps, until your nose is one inch from the floor. Keep your abdominals pulled in tightly and exhale as you push your body weight back to the start position. Repeat for 15 to 25 repetitions. As soon as you complete your repetitions of push-ups, your next step is to immediately hold your weight in a plank position, which is the top of your push-up. If you are doing your push-ups on your knees, lift your knees off the floor and hold your weight with only your toes and hands touching the ground. You are going to feel the work in your chest, shoulders, and triceps. Pull your abdominals in tight to support your lower back, and make sure your back is in a nice straight line. Hold this plank for 30 seconds.

BACK KICK ON FOURS

(Levels 1 to 5; 2- to 10-pound leg weights for Levels 4 and 5)

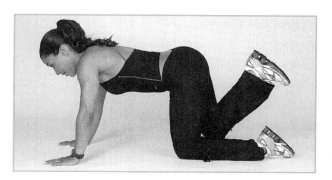 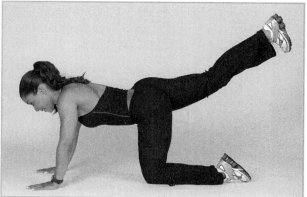

On your hands and knees, create the shape of a box with your body holding your abs tight and back straight. Lift your right knee off the floor and kick your right leg behind you, toward the ceiling at a 45-degree angle, contracting your buttocks (gluteal) muscles. Make sure you keep your abdominals tight to support your lower back. Repeat the back kick motion for 15 to 25 repetitions according to appropriate level. Repeat on your other leg.

• BASIC CRUNCH

(Levels 1 to 5)

Lie on your back, bend your knees, and place your feet on the floor hip distance apart. Place your hands behind your head, pull your navel toward your spine, relax your neck, and make sure there is a space, the size of tennis ball, between your chin and your chest.

Inhale and pull your navel to your spine, contracting your abdominal muscles, then exhale as you lift your head and shoulders off the floor, contracting your abdominal muscles. Hold the crunch at the top for 2 to 3 seconds. Inhale as you slowly return to the starting position for 2 to 3 seconds, but do not release your contraction. Repeat the movement for 15 to 25 repetitions according to your appropriate level, exhaling each time you lift your head and shoulders off the floor. Make sure you feel the contraction in your abdominals each time you lift.

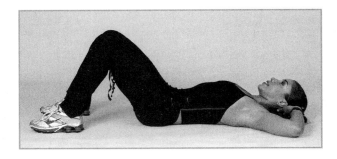

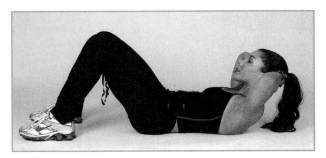

CHEST FLY

(Levels 1 to 5 using 3- to 25-pound dumbbells)

Lie on your back with your knees bent, feet flat on the floor, holding dumbbells with arms extended straight above the shoulders, palms facing each other. Using the muscles in your chest and shoulders, inhale as you slowly open your arms wide, lowering them out and toward the ground. Keep your elbows slightly bent and stop one inch before touching the floor. As you exhale, use your chest and shoulder strength to push the dumbbells back up to the start position. Repeat the movement for 15 to 25 repetitions, according to your appropriate level.

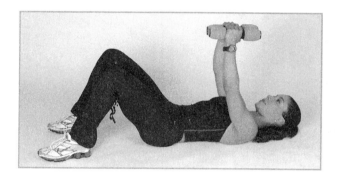

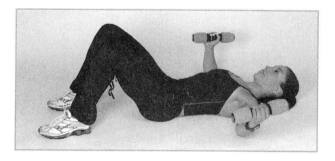

REVERSE LUNGE

(Level 1: Use chair for balance support/Levels 2 to 5: use 5- to 25-pound dumbbells)

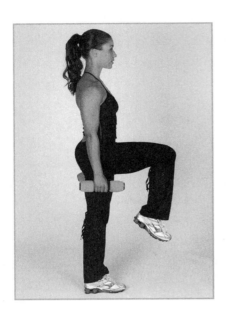
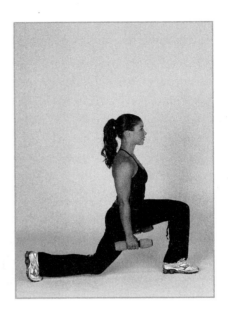

Stand with your legs hip distance apart and feet parallel. Step back with your right leg about 3 to 4 feet (depending on your height), landing on the ball of your foot with your heel off the floor. Slowly lower your body weight down into a lunge. Your front knee should be directly over your heel, creating a 90-degree angle thigh to shin, and the back leg should be straight but not hyperextended. Your back knee should never touch the floor. Over time as you practice and improve you will be able to lower deeper into your lunge. Exhale as you drive your body weight through your left heel and straighten your left leg to a standing position, contracting your left buttocks, quadriceps, and hamstring. At the same time lift your right foot off the floor and your right knee up to hip level. Repeat the movement by stepping back again with the right foot. Inhale as you lower into the reverse lunge and exhale as you push back up to the standing position. If you are doing this exercise with weights, hold them firmly and let your arms drop along the sides of your body but still with some control. Repeat the reverse lunge on the other leg the appropriate number of reps for your level.

• REPEATER KNEE

(Levels 1 to 5)

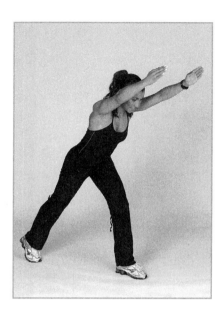 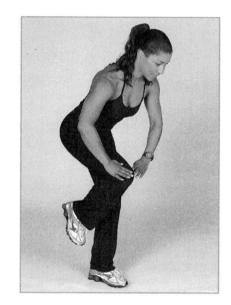

From a standing position with feet parallel and hip distance apart, step your right foot back 3 to 4 feet (depending on your height) and place the ball of your right foot on the floor with the heel elevated. With all of your weight on your left leg, reach both arms overhead toward the ceiling on a diagonal. Your body should create a long line from your fingertips, through your spine, through your right leg all the way to your right toes.

Inhale and pull your navel toward your spine, contracting your abdominal muscles. Exhale as you simultaneously pull your right knee up to your abdominals and bring both arms down to touch the top of your knee. Return to the start position and repeat for 15 to 25 repetitions, according to your appropriate level. Remember to exhale each time you lift your knee. When finished, repeat with the other leg.

• OVERHEAD PRESS

(Levels 1 to 5 using 3- to 25-pound dumbbells)

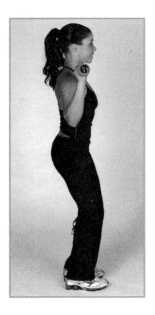 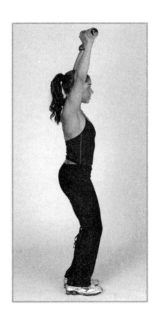

Stand up tall with feet hip width apart, a slight bend in the knees, neck and shoulders relaxed, and abdominal muscles pulled in tight to protect your lower back. Hold the dumbbells one inch above shoulders, with palms facing straight ahead and elbows bent. Inhale and pull your navel toward your spine. Exhale as you press the dumbbells straight overhead until both arms are extended straight, contracting shoulders (deltoids). Be careful not to lock elbows. Return arms to the start position and repeat movement for 1 to 25 repetitions, according to your appropriate level.

SQUAT AND CHAIR POSE

(Levels 1 to 5 using 3- to 25-pound dumbbells)

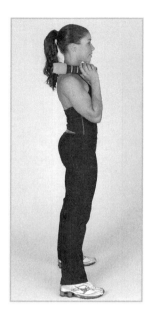 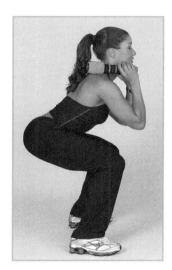 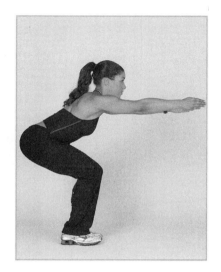

Stand up tall with feet parallel and slightly wider than shoulder width apart. Place dumbbells on top of shoulders and support them with your hands. Inhale as you send your hips behind you as if you are going to sit in a chair. Feel your body weight move into the heels of your feet. To avoid unnecessary stress on your knees, make sure your knees do not push over your toes. Exhale as you push your hips through your heels back up to the standing position, squeezing your buttocks and abdominals when you return to the start position. Repeat the movement for 15 to 25 repetitions, according to your appropriate level. (The chair pose is not demonstrated on the *Hollywood Trainer Weight-Loss Plan Workout* DVD).

At the end of each set of squats, hold an isometric chair pose. Place your feet together, send your hips back into a squat, and stay there as you contract the top of your thighs (quadriceps) for 30 to 60 seconds, according to your appropriate level. As you squat, extend your arms in front of you so they are parallel to the floor. (For an easier option, you can rest your hands lightly on your thighs.) This chair pose can also be done against a wall. Just make sure you use good squat form and keep your knees directly over the toes.

ALTERNATING KNEE-UP

(Levels 1 to 5)

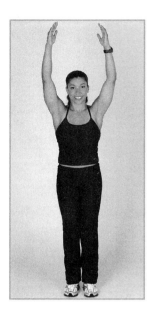 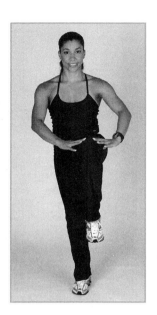

Stand up tall with your feet parallel and hip distance apart. Extend both arms straight overhead. Inhale and contract your abdominals. Exhale as you simultaneously lift your right knee up to your abdominals and pull both arms down and across the torso to touch the top of your right knee. Return to the start position and repeat the movement with the left knee. Continue to alternate the movement from right knee to left knee until you have completed 15 to 25 repetitions on each leg. Remember to exhale and squeeze your abdominals as you raise your knee.

• OVERHEAD TRICEPS EXTENSION

(Levels 3 to 5 using 3- to 25-pound dumbbells)

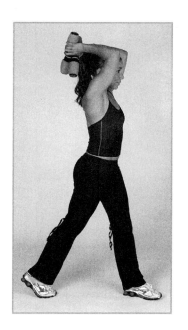 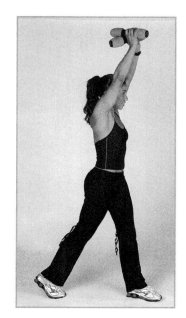

Holding one or two dumbbells in both hands in front of your body, stand tall with feet parallel and hip distance apart. Step the right foot straight back behind you 10 to 12 inches, placing the ball of right foot on the ground to support lower back. Exhale as you contract your abdominals and lift the dumbbell overhead, keeping your elbows bent to 90 degrees and close to your head. At the top of the move, inhale, pull abs in tight to support lower back, then exhale as you press the dumbbell toward the ceiling until arms are straight. Squeeze the back of your arms (triceps), as you press toward the ceiling. As you inhale, slowly lower your forearms, keeping your elbows close to your head. Repeat the movement for 15 to 25 repetitions, according to your appropriate level.

SINGLE LEG REACH

(Levels 3 to 5)

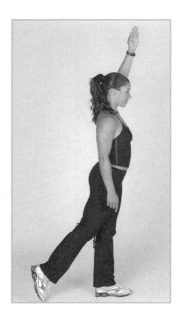 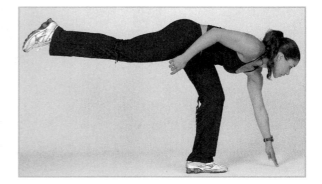

From a standing position with feet parallel and hip width apart, place all of your body weight on your left leg and move your right leg behind you until it is extended straight and on a diagonal with a pointed toe. (Beginners can bend the right leg, resting lightly on the ball of the right foot at the start position.) Balancing on the left leg, inhale and pull your abdominals in tight. Exhale as you reach forward with your right hand and lightly touch the floor. Inhale and pull your abdominals in again, and exhale to return to a standing position on the left leg. Repeat the movement for 10 to 15 repetitions, according to your appropriate level. Remember to keep the abdominals contracted to help you balance and to help support your lower back. Your back should stay straight while you are executing this movement and your back leg should come off the floor so you are balancing all of your weight on one leg. Repeat exercise on your other leg.

STANDING OBLIQUE CRUNCH

(Levels 3 to 5)

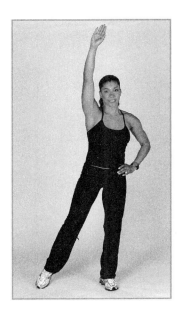 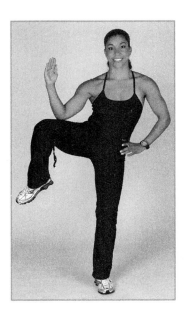

From a standing position with feet parallel and hip width apart, extend your right arm above your head and extend your right leg to the right side of your body. Balance on your left leg. Inhale. Exhale, contracting your obliques and abdominals, as you simultaneously pull your right elbow down and your right knee up until they meet at your side. Repeat for 15 to 25 repetitions, depending on your own level. When finished, repeat the same movements on the other side.

• TRICEPS KICKBACK

(Levels 4 to 5, using 3- to 25-pound dumbbells)

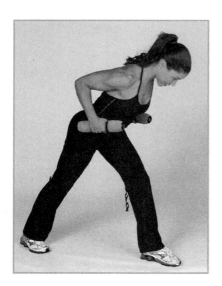 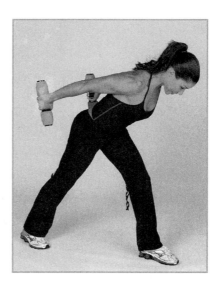

From a standing position with feet parallel and hip width apart, create a two-point stance by placing your right leg about 3 to 4 feet behind you. A nice diagonal line should run from the crown of your head, through your spine, through your right leg all the way to your toes. Holding the dumbbells in each hand, palms facing toward you, keep your arms close to the sides of your torso. You start the movement with your elbows bent. Inhale and pull your abdominals in tight. Exhale as you extend your arms back by pressing the weights behind you until your arms are straight. Do not lock your elbows. Squeeze the backs of your arms (triceps). Inhale as you return to the start position. Repeat the movement for 15 to 25 repetitions, according to your appropriate level. Make sure you feel the contraction in your triceps with each kickback.

• SINGLE LEG SQUAT

(Levels 4 and 5, using 3- to 25-pound dumbbells)

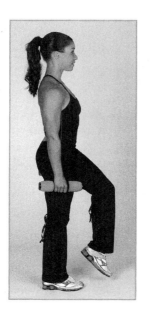 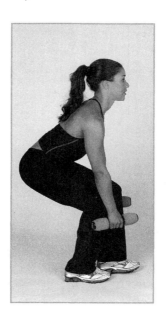

From a standing position with feet parallel and hip width apart, shift all of your body weight onto your right heel. Lift your left heel off the floor so that only your left toes are touching the floor. Inhale and pull your navel toward your spine, exhale, and hold your starting position with tight abdominals. Inhale as you slowly send both hips back, carrying all of your body weight in the right hip, buttocks, quadriceps, and hamstring. Sit back as low as you can without pushing your knee over your toes. Your right knee must stay directly above your right toes. You should not feel any pain or discomfort in your right knee. Exhale and drive through your right heel, contracting your buttocks, quadriceps, and hamstring, and return to the standing position. As you sit back into your single leg squat, the opposite leg just goes along for the ride. With each repetition try to lift the left toes off the floor to make your right side work even more to balance. Repeat the movement 10 to 15 repetitions according to your appropriate level. When finished, repeat the same movements on the other leg.

• CROSS-TORSO REPEATER KNEE

(Levels 4 to 5)

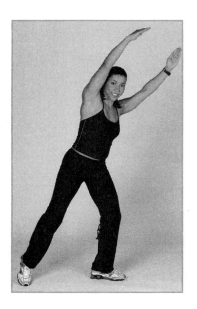 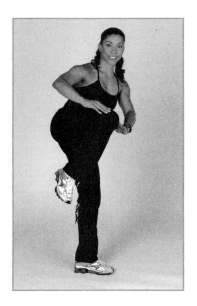

Standing tall with feet parallel and hip width apart, shift all of your body weight onto your left leg and extend your right leg to the right with only your right toes touching the floor. Reach both arms in the air on a diagonal to the left of your body. Your arms and your right leg should create a long diagonal line. Inhale and pull your navel to your spine; exhale as you simultaneously pull your right knee toward your abdominals and both arms down to touch the top of your right knee. Return your arms and right leg to the starting position. The left leg is also working to hold your body weight. Repeat the movement for 1 to 25 repetitions, according to your appropriate level. When finished, repeat the same movements on the other leg.

25

CORE

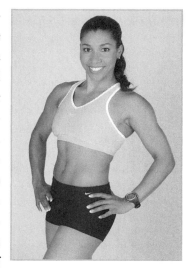

n addition to circuit training and cardio training, I also recommend exercises that strengthen the core muscles in the
abdomen and lower back. We spend roughly $50 billion a
year on the treatment of lower back pain, and it's estimated
that four out of five Americans will have some form of lower
back injury in their lifetime. Most people simply don't understand how important it is to strengthen their core muscles.
You use them every time you stand up, sit down, pick something up, push something overhead, balance, reach from side
to side, stretch overhead, walk, jog, run, hike, bike, climb
stairs, play sports, clean the house, carry groceries . . . basi-
cally every time you move. So quite apart from the obvious
cosmetic benefits of tightening your stomach or getting rid of
those love handles, working your core muscles to make them flexible and strong will help you
enormously in your everyday life and reduce the risk of injury and pain. There are three levels
of the Core Workout. I recommend that you start at Level 1 and then progress to Level 2 after you

can successfully complete all of the repetitions of each exercise with good form and technique and you no longer feel challenged. (To help you learn proper form and technique, I recommend following the Core Workout on *The Hollywood Trainer Weight-Loss Plan Workout* DVD.) The Core Workout series is to be done on Day 2, Day 4, and Day 6.

MYTH: *I just need to lose the weight around my stomach, so I am just going to do stomach exercises.*

MYTH-BUSTER: To lose weight, you have to get all of your muscles moving so that you can burn calories. Doing core training (stomach exercises) alone is not enough to help you lose weight. You have to do cardiovascular or aerobic exercise, total body resistance training, flexibility training, and core training to get the best results in the shortest amount of time. You simply will not burn enough calories to burn the fat off over your stomach by doing only core training (stomach exercises).

THE 7-DAY HOLLYWOOD TRAINER WEIGHT-LOSS PLAN WORKOUT

Day 1: Cardio Burn; Stretch-It-Out
Day 2: Chest, Tri's, and Booty (Circuit A); **Core;** Stretch-It-Out
Day 3: Cardio Burn; Stretch-It-Out (Flexibility Stretching)
Day 4: Back, Bi's, and Thighs (Circuit B); **Core;** Stretch-It-Out
Day 5: Chest, Tri's, and Booty (Circuit A); Stretch-It-Out
Day 6: Back, Bi's, and Thighs (Circuit B); **Core;** Stretch-It-Out
Day 7: Rest, Relax, and Rejuvenate

CORE WORKOUT: LEVEL 1

Listen to your body when executing all of the core exercises. You should not feel any pain in your lower back. Do as many reps as you can sustain with good form and technique, and take a break whenever you need to. Progress slowly, and each time you do the Core Workout, your strength and endurance will improve.

Basic Crunch: 15 reps

Roll-up (with bent knees): 8 reps

Reverse Crunch (with bent knees): 15 reps

Single Oblique Crunch: 15 each side

Boat Pose: 3 sets and hold each for 8 breaths

Side Reach (lying with bent legs): 8 reps

Alternating Leg Lift (with bent knees): 15 reps (*The Hollywood Trainer Weight-Loss Plan Workout* DVD does not have this exercise and instead has an exercise called Alternating Obliques.)

Torpedo Back Extension: 1 set/8 breaths

Superman: 2 sets of 4 reps/8 breaths

Shell Stretch: 3 sets and hold each for 3 to 4 breaths

Cobra Stretch: 3 sets and hold each for 3 to 4 breaths

CORE WORKOUT: LEVEL 2

Now that you are used to the exercises, it's time to take the workout to the next level by increasing the number of repetitions, changing some of the movements to a more advanced option, and adding exercises.

Basic Crunch: 15–25 reps

Roll-up (with straight legs): 8 reps

Reverse Crunch (with straight legs): 15 to 20 reps

Bicycle Crunch: 15 to 20 reps

Boat Pose: 3 sets and hold each for 8 breaths

Side Reach (lying, with lifting leg): 8 reps

Alternating Leg Lift (with straight legs): 15 reps (*The Hollywood Trainer Weight-Loss Plan Workout* DVD does not have this exercise. Instead, it has an exercise called Alternating Obliques.)

Iso-Ab Plank: 3 sets

Torpedo Back Extension with Arms: 1 set/8 reps and 8 breaths

Superman: 2 sets/8 breaths each

Swimming: 2 sets/8 breaths

Shell Stretch: 3 sets for 3 to 4 breaths

Cobra Stretch: 3 sets for 3 to 4 breaths

CORE WORKOUT: LEVEL 3

To challenge your core, and sculpt and define your abdominals, I have increased the number of repetitions, changed some of the movements to a more advanced option, and added some exercises.

Basic Crunch with arm reach: 15–25 reps

Roll-up (with straight legs): 8 reps

Reverse Crunch (with straight legs): 25 reps

Bicycle Crunch: 25 reps

Boat Pose: 3 sets and hold each for 8 breaths

Side Reach (lying, with lifting legs): 8 reps

Alternating Leg Lift (with straight legs): 15 reps (*The Hollywood Trainer Weight-Loss Plan Workout* DVD does not have this exercise. Instead, it has an exercise called Alternating Obliques.)

Double Leg Reach: 8 reps

Iso-ab Plank Combo: 1 set

Torpedo Back Extension with Arms: 1 set of 8 reps and 8 breaths

Superman (simultaneous arms and legs lift): 2 sets/8 breaths each

Swimming: 2 sets, 9 breaths

Shell Stretch: 3 sets, 5 to 6 breaths

Cobra Stretch: 3 sets, 6 to 7 breaths

CORE WORKOUT EXERCISES

• BASIC CRUNCH

(Levels 1 and 2)

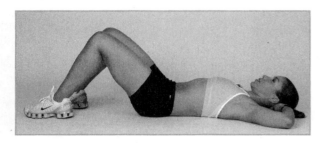

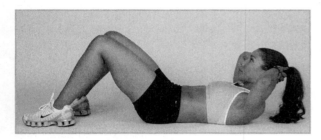

Lie on your back, bend your knees, place your feet on the floor hip distance apart, and place your hands lightly behind your head. Inhale as you pull your navel toward your spine, relax your neck, and make sure there is a space, the size of tennis ball, between your chin and your chest. Exhale and feel yourself contract your abdominals as you lie on your back. Inhale and pull your navel to your spine, contracting your abdominal muscles, then exhale as you lift your head and shoulders off the floor by engaging and contracting your abdominal muscles for 2 to 3 seconds. Do not use your hands and arms to lift yourself—let the abdominals do the work. Inhale as you slowly return to the floor for 2 to 3 seconds but do not release your contraction. Repeat the movement for 15 to 25 repetitions according to your appropriate level. Make sure you feel the contraction in your abdominals each time you lift.

• BASIC CRUNCH (WITH ARM REACH)

(Level 3)

Start with your hands behind your head. Exhale and crunch. Hold your crunch position
and as you inhale, reach your arms in front of
you toward the top of your knees, trying to lift
your chest a little bit higher and feeling more of
a contraction in your abdominals. Holding that
position and the contraction in your abdominals, exhale and reach your arms beside your
ears as you reach your hands toward the ceiling. You should feel more of a challenge in
your upper abdominal fibers as you try to carry
the weight of your arms with your upper abdominal fibers. Return to the start position and
repeat for a total of 15 to 25 repetitions.

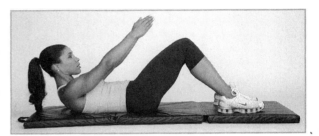

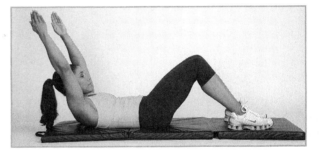

● ROLL-UP (WITH BENT KNEES)

(Level 1)

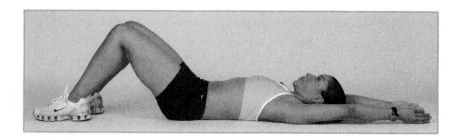

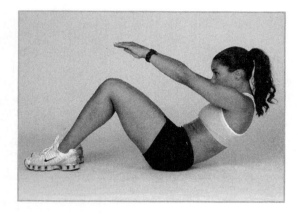

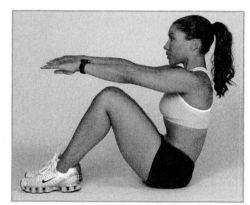

• ROLL-UP (WITH STRAIGHT LEGS)

(Level 2 and 3)

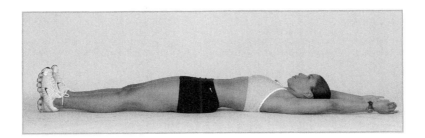

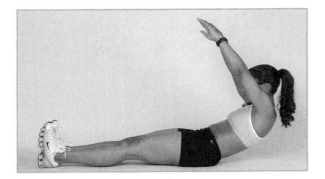

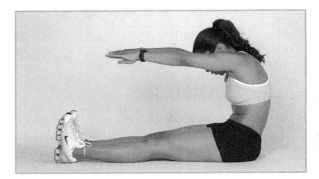

Lie on your back, bend your knees, and place your feet on the floor hip width apart. (Levels 2 and 3: straighten your legs on the floor with your feet flexed and inner thighs touching.) Reach your arms long above your head and extended alongside your ears on the floor, palms facing up. Inhale, pull your navel to your spine, and reach your arms up to the ceiling. Exhale as you contract your abdominals and lift your head, neck, and chest up off the floor, one vertebra at a time, keeping your spine rounded. The point is to move smoothly through this exercise and avoid jerky movements and undue straining.

At the top of the roll-up, inhale and pull your abdominals in tight as you begin to roll back down on the rounded spine. Exhale as you continue to roll back, releasing to the floor one vertebra at a time (lower back, mid-back, upper back). Repeat this complete movement 8 times.

REVERSE CRUNCH (WITH BENT KNEES)

(Level 1)

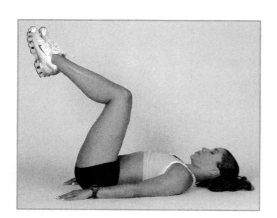 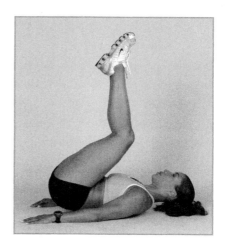

REVERSE CRUNCH (WITH STRAIGHT LEGS)

(Levels 2 and 3)

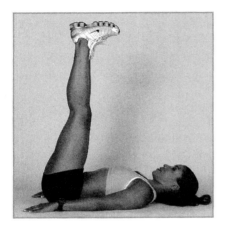 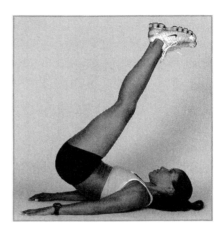

Lie on your back, bend your knees, and lift your feet off the floor, stacking your knees over your hips, keeping your legs close together but not pressing too tightly. (Levels 2 and 3: straighten your legs toward the ceiling, perpendicular to the floor.) Inhale and pull your navel to your spine. Exhale as you contract your lower abdominals to lift your hips gently off the floor. Inhale as you slowly resist and use your lower abdominals to lower your hips back to the floor. Each time you contract your lower abdominals, keep in mind that you are trying to bring your hips (pelvis) closer to your rib cage. Repeat the movement: exhale as you lift the hips, inhale as you return your hips to the floor for 15 to 25 reps according to your appropriate level.

SINGLE OBLIQUE CRUNCH

(Level 1)

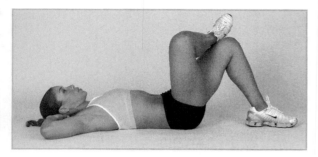

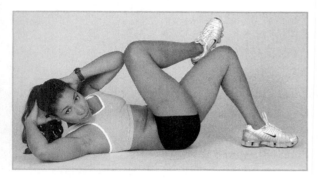

Lie on your back and cross your right ankle over your left thigh. Place your hands loosely behind your head, pull your navel toward your spine, relax your neck, and make sure there is a space the size of a tennis ball between your chin and your chest. Exhale and feel yourself contract your abdominals as you lie on your back.

Inhale and pull your navel to your spine; then, on the exhale, lift your left shoulder off the ground toward your right knee. Feel the contraction in your abdominals and obliques. Return to the start position and repeat until you have completed 15 repetitions, exhaling as you lift off the floor and inhaling as you slowly resist back down. Repeat the movement on the other side.

• BICYCLE CRUNCH

(Levels 2 and 3)

Lie on your back, bend your knees, and lift your feet off the floor, stacking your knees over your hips, keeping your legs as close together as is comfortable but not pressing them together too tightly. Exhale as you bring the left shoulder off the ground and the right knee into the center of your torso. Touch your right knee with your left elbow as you extend your left leg away from your body on a diagonal. Pull your abdominals in tightly, as you need to contract your rectus abdominis, transversus abdominis, and obliques to successfully maximize this movement. Repeat the movement on the other side by touching your left knee with your right elbow as you extend your right leg away from your body on a diagonal. Make sure you keep your lower back in contact with the floor. Continue to repeat this movement, alternating left elbow to right knee and right elbow to left knee.

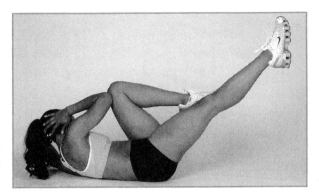

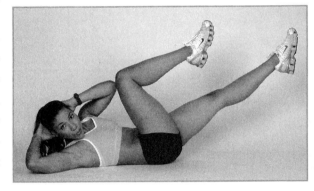

Inhale for one touch on each side (a rotation). Exhale for a rotation. Complete 15 to 25 rotations, according to your appropriate level. Rotating both left and right is considered one rotation.

• BOAT POSE 1

(Level 1)

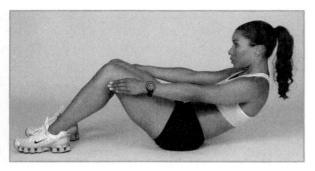

Sit on your buttocks with your knees bent and your feet on the floor hip width apart. Place your hands underneath your thighs, take a deep inhale, and lengthen your spine nice and tall. Exhale and pull your abdominals in tight as you lower halfway to the floor. Release your hands from your thighs and hold this position (isometric rectus abdominis contraction) for 8 full breaths. Each time you exhale feel the contraction in your abdominals. Repeat this exercise for a total of 3 sets.

• BOAT POSE 2

(Level 2)

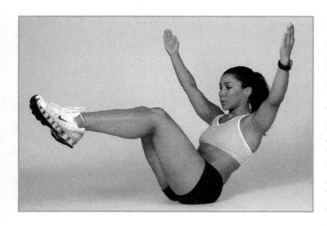

Sit on your buttocks with your knees bent and your feet on the floor hip width apart. Place your hands underneath your thighs, take a deep inhale, and lengthen your spine nice and tall. As you exhale, slowly lift each foot off the floor, keeping your knees bent. You will rock back on your sitz bones, but try to balance without going too far onto the small of your back. Release your grip on your thighs and open your arms wide. Your legs and arms are now acting as additional weight against your abdominals. Hold for 8 full breaths. Repeat this movement for a total of 3 sets.

• BOAT POSE 3

(Level 3)

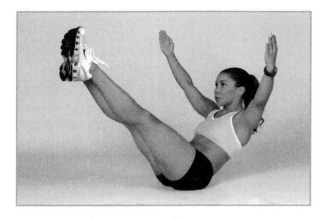

Sit on your buttocks with your knees bent and your feet on the floor hip width apart. Place your hands underneath your thighs, take a deep inhale, and lengthen your spine nice and tall. Inhale and hold. Then as you exhale, slowly lift one foot off the floor, extending the leg until it is straight and on a diagonal. Inhale again, then exhale as you slowly lift the other foot off the floor, extending both legs until they are straight and on a diagonal, balancing on your sitz bones. Release the grip on your thighs, open your arms wide, and hold for 8 full breaths. Repeat this movement for a total of 3 sets.

SIDE REACH (LYING WITH BENT LEGS)

(Level 1)

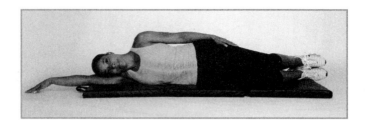

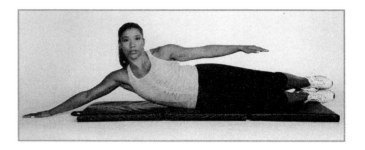

• SIDE REACH (LYING, WITH LIFTING LEGS)

(Levels 2 and 3)

Lie down on your right side with your complete side, head to toe, flush to the mat. Rest your head on your right arm. Pull your knees up toward your chest to create a 90-degree angle of your thighs to your body. (Levels 2 and 3: keep your legs straight and extended long.)

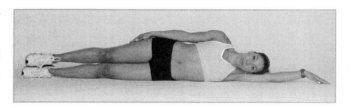

Inhale and pull your navel to your spine; exhale and engage your abdominals and obliques to reach your left arm down your left side as if you are going to touch

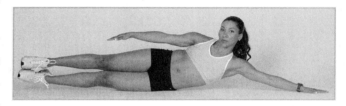

your ankle. You will be lifting only slightly off the floor. Don't strain or jerk to get higher off the floor. Feel your abdominals and obliques contract as you reach down your side. Inhale as you lower yourself, resisting with your abdominals and obliques. Repeat the movement for a total of 8 reps. Complete the exercise with 8 reps on the opposite side.

● ALTERNATING LEG LIFT (WITH BENT KNEES)

(Level 1)

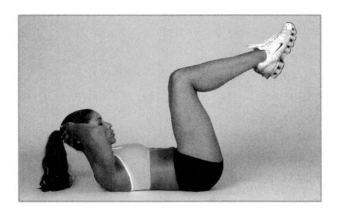

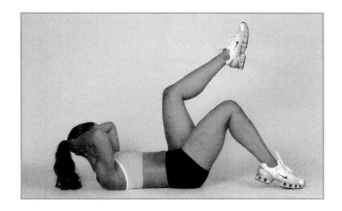

• ALTERNATING LEG LIFT (WITH STRAIGHT LEGS)

(Levels 2 and 3)

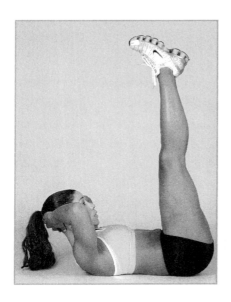
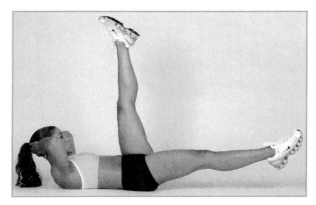

Lie on your back, bend your knees, and lift your feet off the floor, stacking your knees directly over your hips. (Levels 2 and 3: straighten your legs toward the ceiling, perpendicular to the floor.) Make sure your lower back is in contact with the mat and your pelvis is in its neutral position; that is, your pelvis is not tilted front or back. Inhale and pull your navel to your spine; exhale and slowly lower your right foot toward—but not quite touching—the floor. (Level 1: keep the knee bent and let your right foot touch the floor to make the move easier; Levels 2 and 3: keep the leg straight.) Inhale and return the leg to the start position. When the leg is extended away from the body, squeeze your transversus abdominis (deep lower abdominal muscle fibers below your belly button) and your "6-pack" (rectus abdominis). Make sure your lower back remains in contact with the floor. Repeat the movement with the other leg. Exhale as you lower the leg, and inhale as you bring the leg back over the hip. Continue to alternate (right leg exhale down, inhale up; left leg exhale down, inhale up) until you have completed 15 reps on each side. (*The Hollywood Trainer Weight-Loss Plan Workout* DVD does not have this exercise; instead it has an exercise called Alternating Obliques.)

■ DOUBLE LEG REACH

(Level 3)

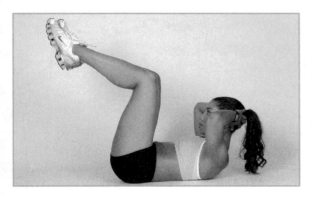

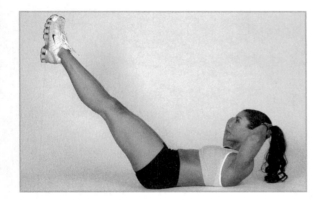

Lie on your back and start in the basic crunch position with your hands behind your head, your knees bent, and your feet flat on the floor. Now lift your feet off the floor and stack your knees over your hips. Make sure your thighs are together and your shins are parallel to the floor. Inhale and pull your navel to your spine, contracting your abdominals; exhale and lift your shoulders off the ground, contracting your abdominals while keeping your knees in the same position stacked over your hips. Inhale again holding this position. Now exhale, pulling your abs in as tightly as you can, and reach both legs away from your body on a diagonal with your thighs together. Make sure your lower back does not lift off the floor. Your legs are acting as a weight on your lower abdominal fibers (transversus abdominis and rectus abdominis). Inhale and bring your knees back over your hips, keeping your head and shoulders off the floor. Exhale and reach the legs out again. Continue to inhale and bring the knees in, and exhale to reach the legs out for a total of 8 reps.

ISO-AB PLANK

(Level 2)

Lie facedown on the mat with your body in a long, straight line, feet flexed, and prop yourself up on your forearms, with your elbows directly underneath your shoulders. Inhale and pull your navel to your spine, squeezing your abs; exhale as you contract your abdominals and lift your hips off the floor as your knees remain on the mat. Make sure your spine is in a nice straight line parallel to the floor. On the next exhale, contract your abdominals to lift your knees off the floor. Continue to pull your abs in tight and try to be as light as you can on your elbows and toes. (Imagine that someone 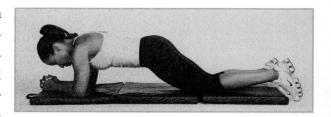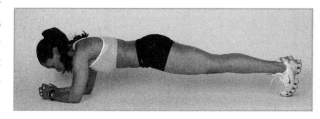 is trying to punch you in the stomach and you must flex your abdominals as tightly as you can to resist the punch.) Continue to inhale and exhale with force, using your abs to carry your body weight. Hold for thirty seconds and then repeat 2 more times.

ISO-AB PLANK (WITH SINGLE ARM/LEG LIFTS)

(Level 3)

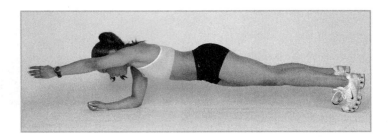

Using the same great Iso-Ab Plank form as described for Level 2, on your next exhale reach your left arm in front of you, which will force you to stabilize on three points (toes and right forearm). Contract your abdominals as tightly as you can to balance and stabilize. Hold for 15 seconds. Replace the left elbow under your shoulder and lift your left leg for 15 seconds, then your right leg, and then your right arm. Hold each limb in the air for 15 seconds, balancing and stabilizing with the strength of your abdominals.

ISO-AB PLANK (WITH SIMULTANEOUS ARM/LEG LIFT)

(Level 3)

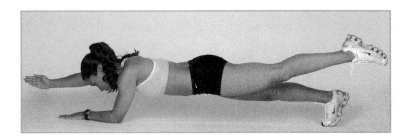

From the Iso-Ab Plank position, reach your right arm *and* your left leg away from your torso, balancing on your left arm and right toes. Contract your abdominals as tightly as you can, continue to breathe, exhaling with force, and hold for 30 seconds.

• TORPEDO BACK EXTENSION

(Level 1)

Lie facedown with arms extended along the body, palms facing in. Inhale and lengthen your body into a nice long line by extending your legs and pointing your toes. Reach your hands strongly toward your toes as you drop your shoulders down and away from your ears, lengthening your neck. (Imagine there is a string attached to the crown of your head and it is pulling your spine in a straight line like the shape of a torpedo.) All of

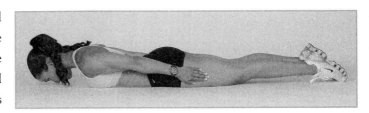

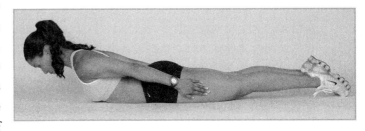

your muscles should be engaged. Continue to lengthen the body; exhale and contract the back muscles that line your spine to lift your chest slightly off the floor, about two inches. Keep a nice long spine and maintain the shape of a torpedo. Hold this position for 8 full breaths.

• TORPEDO BACK EXTENSION

(Levels 2 and 3)

Begin in the Torpedo Back Extension position from Level 1. Inhale and reach both arms forward, creating a "dive" position; exhale and pull your arms back and down to your sides, lifting your chest slightly off the floor, to finish in the long, extended torpedo position. Inhale and dive the arms forward; exhale and pull your arms to your side, slightly lifting your chest off the floor. Repeat the movement 7 times.

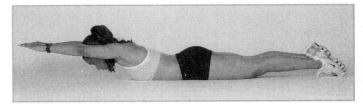

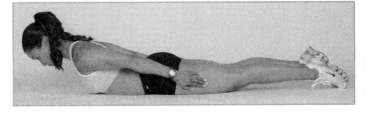

• SUPERMAN

(Level 1)

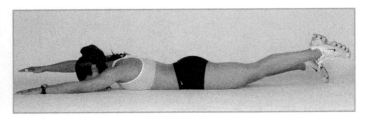

Lie facedown, forehead on the mat and legs straight out and close together in a Superman-flying position with arms extended long, above your head. Inhale and reach through your arms and legs to lengthen your limbs as much as you can; exhale as you lift your right arm and left leg off the floor at the same time as you reach away from your body. Inhale and lower both limbs back to the floor; exhale and lift your left arm and right leg off the floor at the same time, reaching through both limbs, extending the muscles as much as you can. Continue to repeat the movement, alternating sides. Exhale to lift opposite arm and opposite leg; inhale to lower opposite arm and opposite leg until you have repeated each side 4 times. Feel yourself use your back muscles that line your spine. Rest for 30 seconds and then repeat the exercise again.

• SUPERMAN

(Levels 2 and 3)

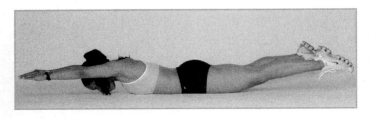

Lie facedown, forehead on the mat and legs straight out and close together in a Superman-flying position with arms extended long, above your head. Exhale and lift both arms and both legs off the floor as if you were flying like Superman. Inhale and hold the position. Exhale and try to reach through your arms and legs, extending and lengthening your muscles. Continue to hold the position by contracting your back muscles for 7 more breaths. Relax for 30 seconds and then repeat the exercise again.

• SWIMMING

(Levels 2 and 3)

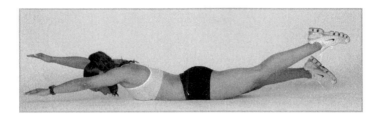

Lie facedown, forehead on the mat and legs straight out and close together in a Superman-flying position, with arms extended long, above your head. Exhale and lift both arms and both legs off the floor as if you were flying like Superman. Inhale and hold the position; exhale and begin pumping both arms and legs as you reach through your limbs. The pumping movement should be up and down, short and controlled. Continue the pumping motion as you inhale and exhale for 8 more breaths.

• SHELL STRETCH

(Levels 1, 2, and 3)

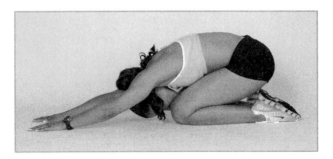

Come onto your hands and knees to create a box shape with your body. Inhale and relax; exhale as you send your hips back to rest your buttocks on your feet as you reach your arms forward on the mat. Hold this position for 5 to 6 breaths, feeling a stretch along your back from your lower back up to your neck.

• COBRA (ABDOMINAL) STRETCH

(Levels 1, 2, and 3)

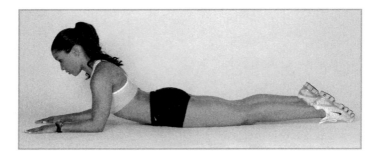

Lie facedown, forehead touching the floor. Place your palms next to your shoulders with your elbows resting close to your torso. Inhale and lengthen your body into a nice long line by pointing your toes, extending—but not lifting—your legs, and lengthening your neck. (Imagine there is a string attached to the crown of your head and it is pulling your spine in a straight line like the shape of a torpedo.) Inhale and exhale two more times, holding this lengthened position. On your next exhale, gently press through the palms of your hands, lifting your chest off the floor. Lift as high as you can without feeling any strain or pain in your lower back. In this Cobra stretch position you should feel a stretch through your abdominals (rectus abdominis). Continue to hold the stretch for 3 to 4 more breaths. Roll down, one vertebra at a time, to the start position. Repeat this total stretch sequence 1 more time.

26

BACK, BI'S, AND THIGHS
(CIRCUIT B)

I n the introduction to the Chest, Tri's, and Booty (Circuit A) there is a description of all of the great benefits of circuit training. The Back, Bi's, and Thighs (Circuit B) is another workout that is in the circuit-training format. This workout is designed to help you burn fat and calories, and sculpt and define your upper back, shoulders, biceps, abdominals, and inner and outer thighs. This particular workout has five levels. I recommend that you start at the first level and then progress to the next level when you can complete all of the exercises with good form and technique and you can complete all of the sets and repetitions required for that level. But listen to your body so that you will instinctively move to the next level

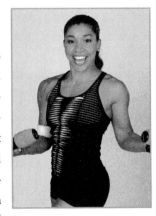

when you feel like you are no longer being challenged. Pull out your Circuit Training Log from your personal journal (Form 9 in the Appendix) and fill in the required information throughout your workout. It is important to record the amount of weight you are using for each specific exercise, the number of repetitions you complete of each movement, and your heart rate at specific points of the workout. All of this information will help you see your progress and decide when it is time to take it to the next level.

> ### THE HOLLYWOOD TRAINER WEIGHT-LOSS PLAN WORKOUT DVD
>
> The Back, Bi's, and Thighs (Circuit B) is included on the DVD. I recommend following it at least the first time through to learn the correct form and technique of each of the exercises. One set of each circuit is performed on the DVD, which is very well organized so that you can complete the exercises for your appropriate level and then repeat them from the top to complete two sets.

Target muscles: back, biceps, shoulders (rear deltoids), inner and outer thighs, and abdominals.

Equipment: dumbbells (beginner: 3 to 5 pounds; intermediate: 5 to 8 pounds; advanced: 5 to 25 pounds), an exercise mat, and a chair (optional to help you balance while doing the Stationary Lunges and Standing Outer Thigh Leg Lifts).

Warm-up and stretch: Start your workout with a 3- to 5-minute warm-up such as power walking, stationary bike, or cardio machine. Complete all of the stretches in the Stretch-It-Out workout, holding each for 8 to 10 seconds.

Exercise Rx: Repeat each circuit twice (2 sets) and then immediately move on to the next. Take a break between exercises and circuits only if you need to. If you complete the specified number of repetitions of an exercise and feel that you can still lift your weight at least 5 more times, you should increase the weight the next time you do the workout. (Remember the Overload principle.)

Cooldown: After you have completed your circuit workout, lower your heart rate by marching on the spot or taking a slow walk for 3 to 5 minutes. Repeat all of the stretches in the Stretch-It-Out workout, holding each stretch for 15 to 30 seconds.

You are required to do the Back, Bi's, and Thighs (Circuit B) on Day 4 and Day 6 of the weekly exercise program.

THE 7-DAY HOLLYWOOD TRAINER WEIGHT-LOSS PLAN WORKOUT

Day 1: Cardio Burn; Stretch-It-Out

Day 2: Chest, Tri's, and Booty (Circuit A); Core; Stretch-It-Out

Day 3: Cardio Burn; Stretch-It-Out (Flexibility Stretching)

Day 4: **Back, Bi's, and Thighs (Circuit B);** Core; Stretch-It-Out

Day 5: Chest, Tri's, and Booty (Circuit A); Stretch-It-Out

Day 6: **Back, Bi's, and Thighs (Circuit B);** Core; Stretch-It-Out

Day 7: Rest, Relax, and Rejuvenate

BACK, BI'S, AND THIGHS (CIRCUIT B) SERIES: LEVEL 1

Complete 2 sets of each circuit.

CIRCUIT 1	15 back flys
	15 plié squats
	15 alternating knee-ups
CIRCUIT 2	15 back rows
	10 stationary lunges (with chair support)
	Lateral side shuffles, 6 reps in each direction
CIRCUIT 3	15 upright rows
	15 standing outer thigh leg lifts (with chair support)
	Touch-heel repeater knees, 25 reps each leg

BACK, BI'S, AND THIGHS (CIRCUIT B) SERIES: LEVEL 2

Just as in the Chest, Tri's, and Booty (Circuit A), Level 2 of Circuit B increases reps and adds drop sets—this time you will be performing drop sets of back flys, back rows, and upright rows.

Complete 2 sets of each circuit.

CIRCUIT 1	Drop set back flys: 15 reps max weight; drop weight 25–50% for 10 more reps.
	15 plié squats
	20 alternating knee-ups
CIRCUIT 2	Drop set back rows: 15 reps max weight; drop weight 25–50% for 10 more reps.
	15 stationary lunges
	Lateral side shuffles: 8 reps each direction
CIRCUIT 3	Drop set upright rows: 15 reps max weight; drop weight 25–50% for 10 more reps.
	25 standing outer thigh leg lifts
	Touch-heel repeater knees: 25 reps each leg

BACK, BI'S, AND THIGHS (CIRCUIT B) SERIES: LEVEL 3

Level 3 adds a fourth circuit and more repetitions to some of the exercises.

Complete 2 sets of each circuit.

CIRCUIT 1	Drop set back flys: 15 reps max weight; drop weight 25–50% for 10 more reps. 25 plié squats 20 alternating knee-ups
CIRCUIT 2	Drop set back rows: 15 reps max weight; drop weight 25–50% for 10 more reps. 15 stationary lunges Lateral side shuffles: 8 reps in each direction
CIRCUIT 3	Drop set upright rows: 15 reps max weight; drop weight 25–50% for 10 more reps. 25 standing outer thigh leg lifts Touch-heel repeater knees: 25 reps each leg
CIRCUIT 4	15 bicep curls 15 standing inner thigh leg lifts 15 standing oblique crunches

BACK, BI'S, AND THIGHS (CIRCUIT B) SERIES: LEVEL 4

This level adds an additional circuit, which means three more exercises, plus additional repetitions for some of the exercises.

Complete 2 sets of each circuit.

CIRCUIT 1	Drop set back flys: 15 reps max weight; drop weight 25–50% for 10 more reps. 25 plié squats 20 alternating knee-ups
CIRCUIT 2	Drop set back rows: 15 reps max weight; drop weight 25–50% for 10 more reps. 15 stationary lunges Lateral side shuffles: 8 reps in each direction
CIRCUIT 3	Drop set upright rows: 15 reps max weight; drop weight 25–50% for 10 more reps. 25 standing outer thigh leg lifts Touch-heel repeater knees: 25 reps each leg
CIRCUIT 4	Drop set 15 bicep curls max weight; drop weight 25–50% for 10 more reps. 25 standing inner thigh leg lifts 25 standing oblique crunches
CIRCUIT 5	External rotation and reach: 10 reps 15 cross-torso repeater knees 15 leg scissors

BACK, BI'S, AND THIGHS (CIRCUIT B) SERIES: LEVEL 5

Congratulations! You've achieved an advanced level of fitness. You should be feeling great. This level adds more repetitions to some of the exercises.

Complete 2 sets of each circuit.

CIRCUIT 1	Drop set back flys: 15 reps max weight, drop weight 25–50% for 10 more reps. 25 plié squats 20 alternating knee-ups
CIRCUIT 2	Drop set back rows: 15 reps max weight; drop weight 25–50% for 10 more reps. 25 stationary lunges Lateral side shuffles: 10 reps in each direction
CIRCUIT 3	Drop set upright rows: 15 reps max weight; drop weight 25–50% for 10 more reps. 25 standing outer thigh leg lifts Touch-heel repeater knees: 25 reps each leg
CIRCUIT 4	Drop set 15 bicep curls max weight; drop weight 25–50% for 10 more reps. 25 standing inner thigh leg lifts 25 standing oblique crunches
CIRCUIT 5	External rotation and reach: 15 reps 25 cross-torso repeater knees 25 leg scissors

BACK, BI'S, AND THIGHS (CIRCUIT B) EXERCISES

• BACK FLY

(Levels 1 to 5, using 3- to 25-pound dumbbells)

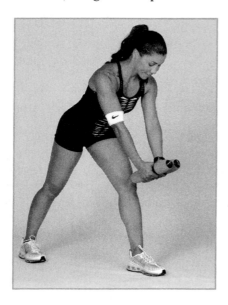 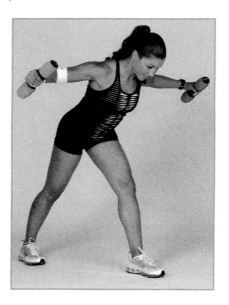

Starting from a standing position with feet parallel and hip width apart, create a two-point stance by placing your right leg behind you about 3 to 4 feet. A nice diagonal line should run from the crown of your head, through your spine, through your right leg, all the way to your toes. Holding on to the dumbbells, palms facing inward, extend both arms toward the ground on a diagonal just in front of your left knee. Inhale and pull your navel to your spine; exhale as you open your arms straight out and toward the ceiling, contracting the muscles in your upper back. Inhale as you slowly lower the weights. Repeat this movement for 15 to 25 repetitions. Keep your neck relaxed and your shoulders down and away from your ears.

PLIÉ SQUAT

(Levels 1 to 5, using 3- to 25-pound dumbbells)

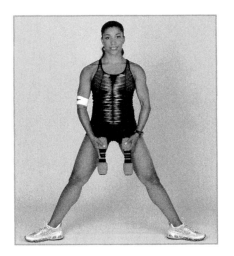 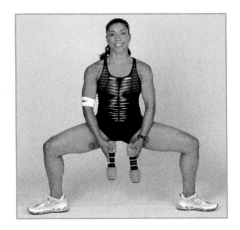

From a standing position, place both feet slightly wider than your shoulders in a turned-out position. (This is also known as second position in ballet.) Hold the dumbbells firmly on top of your shoulders or between your thighs. Inhale as you pull your abdominals in tight and slowly lower your hips toward the floor by bending your knees. Keep your back up nice and tall and imagine that you are sliding your back down a wall. Exhale as you press back to the start position, contracting your buttocks (gluteals) and thighs (adductors). Repeat this movement for 15 to 25 repetitions.

● ALTERNATING KNEE-UP

(Levels 1 to 5)

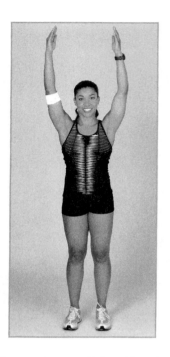 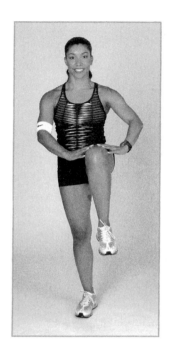

Standing tall with your feet parallel and hip distance apart, extend both arms straight overhead. Inhale and contract your abdominals; exhale as you simultaneously lift your left knee up to your abdominals and pull both arms down and across the torso to touch the top of your left knee. Return to the start position and repeat the movement with the right knee. Continue to alternate the movement from left knee to right knee until you have completed 15 to 25 repetitions on each leg. Remember to exhale and squeeze your abdominals as you raise your knee.

• BACK ROW

(Levels 1 to 5, using 3- to 25-pound dumbbells)

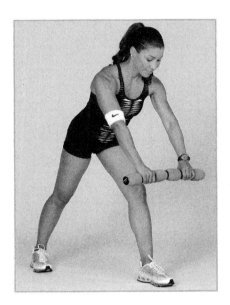 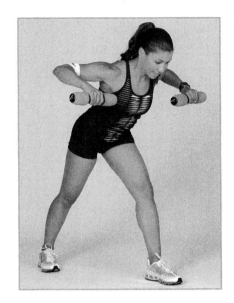

From a standing position with your feet parallel and hip width apart, create a two-point stance by placing your right leg behind you about three to four feet. A nice diagonal line should run from the crown of your head, through your spine, through your right leg, all the way to your toes. Holding on to the dumbbells, palms inward, extend both arms toward the ground just in front of the left knee.

Inhale and contract your abdominals; exhale as you pull your elbows up and back toward the ceiling, bringing the dumbbells to your shoulders and contracting your upper back (rhomboids and latissimus dorsi), biceps, and shoulders. Inhale and lower the weights back to the starting position. Repeat the movements for 15 to 25 repetitions, according to your appropriate level.

STATIONARY LUNGE

(Levels 1 to 5, using 3- to 25-pound dumbbells)

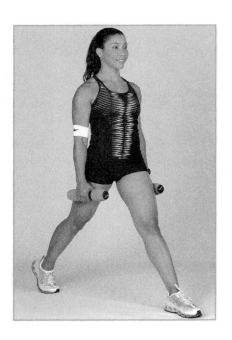 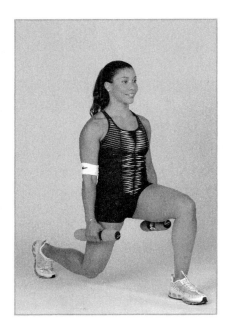

Standing tall with your feet parallel and hip width apart, step your right leg behind you 3 to 4 feet and secure your balance on your right forefoot, keeping your right heel off the ground. Hold dumbbells, palms facing inward, at your sides. (Beginners can do this move without dumbbells and hold onto a secure chair to help with balance.) Inhale and pull your abs in tight; exhale and hold your position. Inhale as you slowly lower your back knee toward the floor, bending your front knee to make a 90-degree thigh-to-shin angle. (If you cannot go to a 90-degree angle, that's okay; you will improve with commitment and consistency.) Make sure your front knee does not push beyond your front toes. Exhale as you push into your left heel and right forefoot until you are standing again and both legs are extended straight. Repeat the movement for 15 to 25 repetitions. Repeat the complete exercise on the opposite leg.

● LATERAL SIDE SHUFFLE

(Levels 1 to 5)

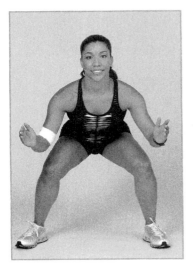 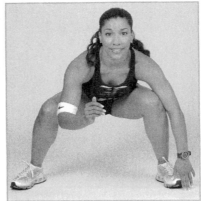 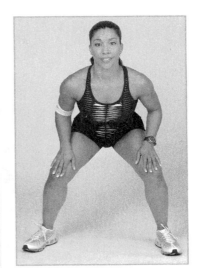

Standing tall with your feet slightly wider than shoulder width apart, send your hips back into a squat position with hands approximately chest height and elbows slightly bent. Shuffle to the left three times and lightly touch the floor with your left hand. (Beginners can touch the top of the thighs with both hands instead of touching the floor). Shuffle three times to the right and touch the floor with the right hand. Continue shuffling from left to right until you have completed 6 to 8 repetitions in each direction, according to your appropriate level.

UPRIGHT ROW

(Levels 1 to 5, using 3- to 25-pound dumbbells)

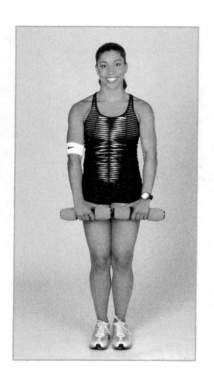 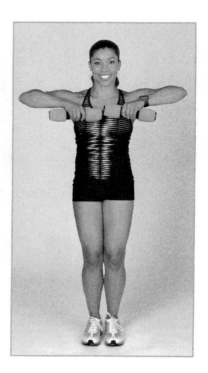

Standing tall with feet hip width apart and holding dumbbells resting on the front of your thighs, press your shoulders down and lengthen your neck. Inhale and contract your abdominals; exhale as you pull the dumbbells up the front of your body to the top of your chest, contracting your shoulders and biceps. Inhale to lower the weights back down. Make sure your elbows are high when pulling the dumbbells up, but keep your neck and shoulders relaxed.

STANDING OUTER THIGH LEG LIFT

(Levels 1 to 5, using zero to 10-pound leg weights)

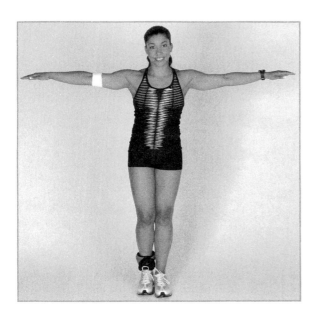 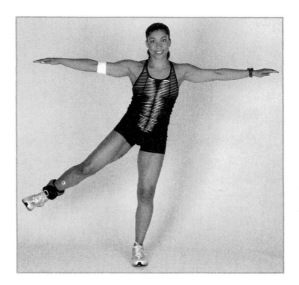

Standing tall with feet parallel and hip width apart, shift your body weight to your left leg. Inhale and pull your navel to your spine; exhale as you open your right leg to the right (abduction), squeezing your outer thigh and buttocks. Inhale and slowly lower your leg back to your starting position. Remember to pull your abdominals in tight to help you balance and support your lower back. Repeat the movement for 15 to 25 repetitions, according to your appropriate level.

Beginners can use a chair for balance and support. And remember to increase the leg weight as you feel up to the challenge.

• TOUCH-HEEL REPEATER KNEE

(Levels 1 to 5)

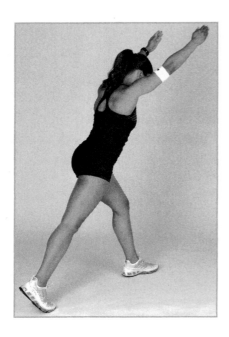 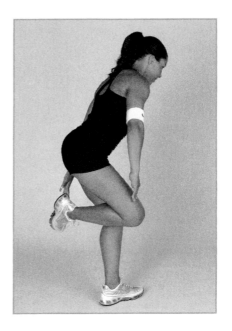

From a standing position with feet parallel and hip width apart, step your right foot behind you 3 to 4 feet, placing the ball of your right foot on the floor with your right heel elevated. Carrying all of your body weight on your left leg, reach both arms overhead toward the ceiling to create a diagonal with your body and your right leg. Inhale and pull your navel toward your spine, contracting your abdominal muscles; exhale as you simultaneously pull your right knee up to your abdominals and both arms down. Touch your right heel with your left hand, contracting your inner thigh muscles (adductors). Remember to exhale each time you touch your heel. Return to the start position and repeat for 15 to 25 repetitions, according to your appropriate level. Repeat the same movements on the other leg.

BICEP CURL

(Levels 3 to 5, using 3- to 25-pound dumbbells)

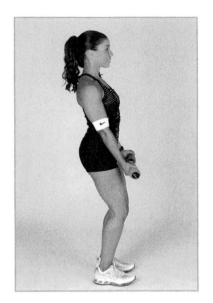 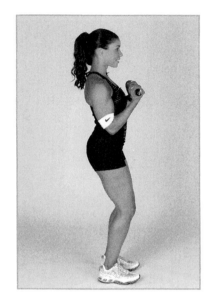

Standing tall with feet hip width apart and knees slightly bent, grasp a dumbbell in each hand with your arms extended downward and palms up. Inhale and pull your navel to your spine. With your upper arms tight against your body, exhale as you bend your elbows and raise the dumbbells up to your shoulders, contracting your biceps. Inhale as you slowly lower the weights. Repeat this movement for 15 to 25 repetitions, according to your appropriate level.

STANDING INNER THIGH LEG LIFT

(Levels 3 to 5, using 0- to 10-pound leg weights)

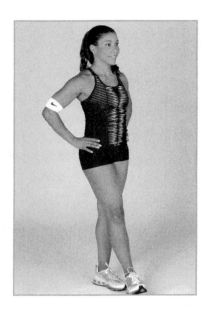 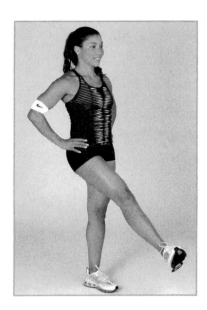

Standing tall, place your right heel directly in front of and at a right angle to your left foot so that your right inner thigh faces forward (away from your body). Your right leg should be externally rotated. Inhale as you pull your abs in tight and elongate your spine; exhale and press your right heel forward until your right foot is about 2 to 3 feet off the ground, squeezing your right inner thigh. Repeat this inner thigh pressing movement for 15 to 25 repetitions, according to your appropriate level. Exhale each time you press the right heel forward. Your abdominals and left leg should always be able to help you balance, stabilize, and hold your position with good form. Repeat the complete exercise with the opposite leg.

STANDING OBLIQUE CRUNCH

(Levels 3 to 5)

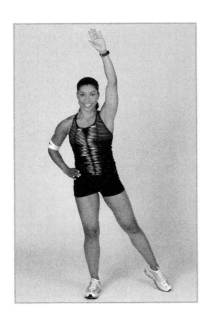 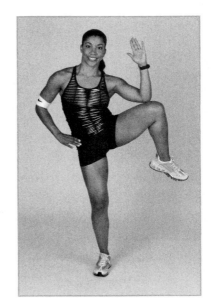

Standing tall with feet parallel and hip width apart, extend your left arm above your head and extend your left leg to the left side of your body, balancing all of your body weight on your right leg. Inhale and contract your abdominals; exhale as you simultaneously pull your left elbow down and your left knee up until they meet at the height of your abdominals, contracting your obliques and abdominals. Repeat this movement for 15 to 25 repetitions. When finished, repeat the same movement on the other side.

• EXTERNAL ROTATION AND REACH

(Levels 4 and 5, using 3- to 10-pound dumbbells)

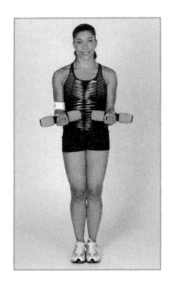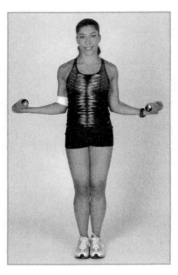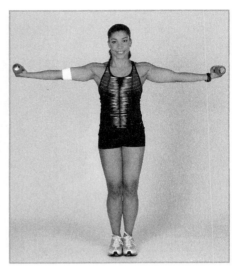

Standing tall with feet hip width apart and knees slightly bent, hold the dumbbells with palms facing the ceiling and elbows bent at 90 degrees, tight to your sides.

Inhale and pull your navel toward your spine, contracting your abdominals; exhale and hold this position. Inhale and externally rotate arms with palms face up, contracting your upper back muscles, keeping your elbows beside your torso. Exhale as you reach your arms away from your body to shoulder height, making the shape of the letter T with your arms and body. Inhale as you lower the weights and return the elbows to your torso. Exhale and internally rotate your arms back to the start position. Repeat this movement for 10 to 15 repetitions, according to your appropriate level.

CROSS-TORSO REPEATER KNEE

(Levels 4 and 5)

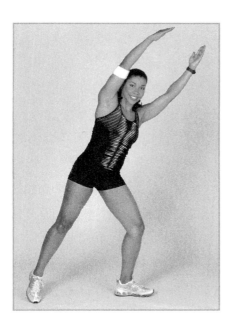 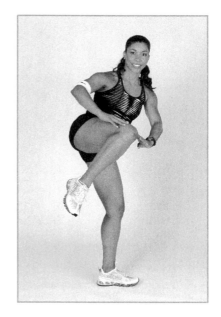

Standing tall with feet parallel and hip width apart, shift all of your body weight onto your left leg, extending your right leg to the right of your body with only your right toes touching the floor. Reach both arms in the air on a diagonal to the left of your body. Your arms and your right leg should create a long diagonal line. Inhale and pull your navel to your spine; exhale as you simultaneously pull your right knee toward your abdominals and both arms down to touch the top of your right knee. Return the arms and right leg to the starting position. (The left leg may bend somewhat at the knee but should always be engaged to help maintain your balance.) Repeat the movement for 15 to 25 repetitions, according to your appropriate level. When finished, repeat the same movements with the other leg.

LEG SCISSOR

(Levels 4 and 5)

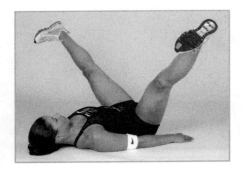 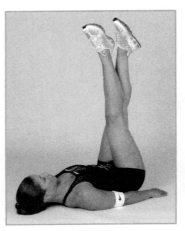 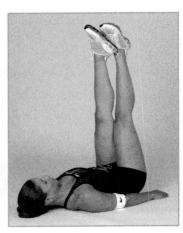

Lie on your back on a mat or towel and extend your legs straight up over your hips. Your legs should be perpendicular to the ground. Inhale and pull your navel to your spine, to support your lower back and the weight of your legs; exhale as you point your feet while pressing energy through your legs, extending them as long as you can. Inhale as you flex your feet and open your legs as wide as you can, lengthening your inner thighs; exhale as you bring your legs together, point your feet, squeezing the inner thighs, cross the right leg over the left, and then the left leg over the right. Try to keep the crisscross movement of the legs small, quick, and controlled. Repeat this movement by opening the legs again on an inhale and then exhale as you crisscross the legs. Inhale to open with feet flexed and exhale to crisscross with pointed feet. Repeat the movement for 15 to 25 repetitions, according to your appropriate level.

27

BEYOND THE HOLLYWOOD TRAINER™ WEIGHT-LOSS PLAN WORKOUT

Once you've made your way through the progressive levels of my program, you have to keep the ball rolling by making exercise fun and exciting. Try new methods like training for a five-kilometer or a minitriathlon. Try some fun classes like Bosu ball, hip-hop dance, salsa, or swing. Get the whole family involved with canoeing, hiking, or skiing. There are several methods of training that you can use to work the four components of fitness—cardiorespiratory fitness, muscular strength, muscular endurance, and flexibility—apart from just training in the gym. Some of the current popular methods of training are yoga, Pilates, Bosu ball, step aerobics, dance aerobics, kickboxing, Swiss ball workouts, medicine ball workouts, indoor cycling, swimming, aqua aerobics, and, of course, sports like basketball, volleyball, hockey, racquetball, and tennis.

Since yoga and Pilates are two of the most popular methods of training that people want to try, and which I especially recommend to all my clients, I've provided you with more information about both of these practices to help you make the right choices when looking for a class or instruction.

YOGA

Yoga is perhaps the most ancient form of exercise that we still do today. There are many different kinds of yoga, but in general yoga practice focuses on the connection between your physical and mental state. Through slow, controlled movements, and concentrating on breath and muscle use, yoga can help you center your energies and reconnect with your body. When practiced over time, it can release accumulated tensions in the body, calm frayed nerves, restructure your spinal alignment, detoxify the blood, increase oxygen absorption (which aids in fat burning!), change brain patterns, and increase happiness through improved hormonal circulation.

When people talk about yoga, they are usually talking about hatha, which exploded in popularity in the United States in the 1960s, almost one thousand years after its creation. It remains the most popular form of yoga practiced in the West. Hatha yoga involves moving through a series of poses, or asanas, that involve breath control, mental focus, and spiritual awareness. Being the oldest form of yoga, hatha has many offshoots, and over the years yogis have developed their own styles and emphases. Some of the more popular forms include Iyengar, which focuses on alignment and posture; Ashtanga, a more athletic form of yoga, involving continuous breath and movement through positions that are held for a short time; and Bikram, developed as a curative measure against injury and done in a heated room, focusing on continuous movement through twenty-six poses. Kundalini yoga, which has been practiced in the West only relatively recently, has a decidedly spiritual emphasis and focuses on awakening inner wisdom through breathing, chanting, and meditation.

Incorporating muscular strength, muscular endurance, flexibility, physical control, breathing, and mental strength, yoga is one of the most complete forms of exercise available. I recommend it highly to anyone at almost any fitness level who's ready to try something a bit different.

There are a couple of things you should keep in mind. The first is that doing yoga means you have to maneuver your body weight through multiple positions. This makes yoga hard for people who are significantly overweight, as they are not strong enough to support their own body weight. If you try to practice yoga before you're ready, you may have a negative experience, or even hurt yourself. If you are significantly overweight I recommend losing weight on my program before starting a yoga class. Also, many people who thrive in high-energy settings with the music pumping may think of yoga as a relatively low-energy, contemplative practice. But you'd be amazed at the different kinds of energy that will be released within the channels of your body—not to mention all the positive results you will see. Although yoga is not a specifically cardiovascular activity, it can absolutely help you lose weight when combined with a cardio training program. Practicing yoga improves your muscular strength and muscular endurance, yet it is very different from traditional weight training because it *lengthens* your muscles while strengthening them, as opposed to shortening them, which is what happens when you train with weights. The result is longer, leaner muscle, and a longer, leaner you. Yoga will also help you manage your stress level, making your cortisol and serotonin release more efficient—another hormonal helper, which means you burn more fat and lose more weight.

If you're a beginner interested in learning yoga, classes are offered at most gyms and health centers, and you can also look for a yoga studio in your area. Group classes are usually relatively inexpensive, although if you are a first-timer I strongly suggest putting a little extra money into a few private sessions, just so you can get some of the basic moves and poses down. There is also a wealth of yoga DVDs and books on the market. But it's best to have some personal instruction so you are starting out on the right track.

PILATES

Joseph Pilates was working as a nurse in England during the 1918 influenza pandemic and looking for a way to rehabilitate bedridden patients. He devised a series of movements that could be practiced within a confined environment, but that effected total body conditioning, increasing flexibility, strength, muscle tone, body awareness, energy, and mental concentration. Rather than performing many repetitions of each exercise, Pilates involves fewer, more precisely controlled movements. Today there are commonly two kinds of Pilates offered in gyms and health centers: mat work, which entails a series of calisthenic motions performed without weights or apparatus, and apparatus work, which requires the use of specially designed machines. Both forms focus on the core postural muscles that keep the body balanced and the spine supported, the theory being that once you strengthen yourself at the core, the rest of your body will move more freely and you will be less susceptible to muscle, joint, and bone problems.

PILATES FOR WEIGHT LOSS?

Pilates will definitely help you lose weight but only when combined with a strength and cardio training program and proper nutrition. Pilates on its own has minimal weight-loss and fat-burning benefits, although it does help you tone your muscles and improve the quality and range of your movement, which in turn increases the effectiveness of your workouts. Keep in mind that many of the Pilates exercises are difficult for overweight people to execute. Because the program emphasizes a focused and controlled use of one's own body weight, it can be hard for heavier people, especially those who carry a lot of extra weight around the abdomen. If you are significantly overweight, I recommend losing weight on my program before trying Pilates. The best way to start doing Pilates is with one or two private sessions so that you can really learn the moves and get the technique down; precision is everything when it comes to Pilates, and it's worth paying a little extra at the beginning to ensure that you will reap all the benefits Pilates has to offer. Having become increasingly popular over the past five years, Pilates classes and instruction are offered at many gyms and physical therapy centers. I particularly recommend the Stott Method of Pilates; Stott has trained Pilates instructors all over the world, and also has an extensive DVD library at www.stottpilates.com.

Part Six

HEALTHY HABITS

FOR LIFE

This section will review the seven simple steps for healthy living so you can continue to incorporate them into your life. Remember that it is the sum of all the steps that will provide you a holistic healthy life. It is just as important that you take a moment to journal your thoughts and watch a beautiful sunset as it is to wake up and start your day with a workout. Don't sweat the small stuff; have fun trying new recipes, new foods, and new activities. Slow and steady wins the race, so always keep in mind that you're only human. You will have tough days, good days, and great days, but don't ever become defeated. Stay on course and stay committed to your journey. There will always be a new sunrise tomorrow. Have faith, believe in yourself, and build a community of friends and family that will support your new lifestyle.

28

21 DAYS AND COUNTING . . .

Congratulations! You have successfully completed the twenty-one days of the Holly-wood Trainer Weight-Loss Plan. Over the course of the past three weeks, you've assessed your mental, spiritual, and physical health and have learned invaluable information about how to get healthy and stay that way for a lifetime. So whether you know it or not, you now have the knowledge and strength to achieve the unique goals you have set for yourself at the beginning of this program.

Now it's time to take all you've learned and apply it to your everyday life as you move beyond my twenty-one-day program.

Remember the Star for Healthy Living, and the seven key principles of health that it represents? In addition to restating these principles below, I have also included additional information and resources, so take the time to review each and be sure you are incorporating them into your life from now on.

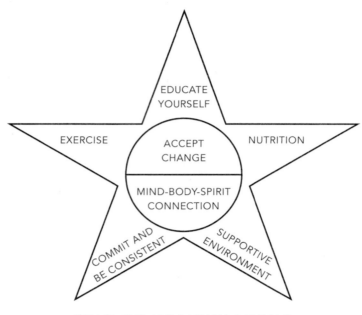

STAR OF HEALTHY LIVING

1. ACCEPT CHANGE

Change is scary for all of us, but now that you've been through my program, you know that change can be good, even great. As you move forward, remember the lessons you've learned over the course of your transformation so far: in order to change the big picture of your life, you have to start with changing the choices you make every single day. At every moment you have the choice to approach a situation with a positive attitude and open heart. Once you start seeing the glass as half full rather than half empty, you'll eliminate unnecessary stress and negativity from your life and your body, and instead open yourself up to the positivity and blessings the universe offers all of us.

2. MAKE THE MIND, BODY, AND SPIRIT CONNECTION

Men often become what they believe themselves to be. If I believe I cannot do something, it makes me incapable of doing it. But when I believe I can, then I acquire the ability to do it even if I didn't have it in the beginning.

—*Mahatma Gandhi*

Doing what's right for your body always starts with your head. In order to enjoy the benefits of the commitment you made during the last three weeks for the rest of your life, you've got to keep the connection between your spirit and your body strong and true. Here are some suggestions for things that you can do on a daily or weekly basis, to keep your mind and body connected and focused:

- Take a little time out from your hectic life to be still and think about where you are in the present moment, where you've been in the past, and where you want to be in the future. Create a space in your home, office, or garden that you can use exclusively for relaxing, meditating, and reflecting. The size of the space is unimportant—what matters is that it's somewhere you feel safe, comfortable, and removed from the hustle and bustle of life. Make use of incense, candles, soothing music, nature sounds, plants, pictures, colors, soft fabrics, and pillows—anything that helps you relax and reflect.

- Get closer to nature: go for walks in whatever open spaces your area has to offer. From the mountains to the valleys (as the song goes) there's some beautiful country out there, and getting out into it will soothe the soul and act as a balm against life's hectic pace.

- For a change of pace—and to get outside your comfort zone—try some form of Eastern exercise: yoga, tai chi, qi gong, meditation, or breathing techniques. There are classes available almost everywhere and audiotapes or DVDs for the novice. These practices are designed to strengthen the mind-body connection.

- Go to your church, temple, mosque, or other place of worship on a regular basis. Stay in touch with your spiritual needs, and your body will thank you.

- Keep up with your journaling. Now that you've completed the twenty-one days of the Hollywood Trainer Weight-Loss Workout Program, you need to stay organized. But, more important, you need to stay accountable for your behavior. You can pay a personal trainer hundreds of dollars, but at the end of the day the only person to whom you have to answer is yourself. Your journal will help you stay the course as well as keep all your activities and records organized. When negative thoughts or energies arise, writing them down is the first step toward resolving them. When positive thoughts arise, write them down too, so you can reflect on them and carry inspiration forward. You can change your approach to or perception of any problem and transform negative situations into positive ones by writing through them. Above all, a strong mind-body connection will help you continue to believe in yourself and your ability to succeed . . . and keep succeeding.

3. EXERCISE: YOU HAVE TO MOVE IT TO LOSE IT!

Now that you've completed the twenty-one days of workouts, it's important to stay committed to working out 4 to 6 times a week for 30- to 60-minute sessions. Your weekly program should include all the components of fitness: cardiorespiratory health, muscular strength, muscular endurance, and flexibility. Each workout should include total body stretches in the warm-up and cooldown, and remember to dedicate time for a deep stretch at least once a week to keep improving your flexibility. You can continue to follow and adapt the seven-day program outlined in Part 4. I provided you with all of those levels so you can stay on the program for an entire year. Be consistent and keep striving for the next level. Post your workout schedule on your fridge, in your daily agenda, on your calendar, and on your computer so you don't forget to schedule workouts into your life. Your health is just as important as your business meetings, hair appointment, picking up the kids, and watching your favorite television show.

THE 7-DAY HOLLYWOOD TRAINER WEIGHT-LOSS PLAN WORKOUT

Day 1: Cardio Burn; Stretch-It-Out

Day 2: Chest, Tri's, and Booty (Circuit A); Core; Stretch-It-Out

Day 3: Cardio Burn; Stretch-It-Out

Day 4: Back, Bi's, and Thighs (Circuit B); Core; Stretch-It-Out

Day 5: Chest, Tri's, and Booty (Circuit A); Stretch-It-Out

Day 6: Back, Bi's, and Thighs (Circuit B); Core; Stretch-It-Out

Day 7: Rest, Relax, and Rejuvenate

When you are able to complete the most-advanced levels, you'll be knowledgeable enough to use my workouts as a template to design your own. There are a lot of exercises to choose from, and you should tailor your workouts to your personal preferences so that they remain enjoyable, challenging, and effective for years to come.

After every four to six weeks of regular training, reassess your workout. Make sure that you are still feeling challenged at the end of every session and that you are giving it 110 percent every time. If you finish a workout and feel like you could keep going, whether it's lifting that weight a few more times or staying on the treadmill for another ten minutes, you need to step it up to prevent your routine from plateauing.

Once you feel comfortable with the form and technique of the exercises in my program, you can start trying new methods of training. For example, you can replace one of the weekly circuit workouts with a boot camp, weight training, kickboxing, or power yoga class. You can replace the flexibility workout with a Pilates or gentle yoga class, or one of the cardio workouts with indoor/ outdoor cycling, the elliptical machine, hiking, swimming, aerobic dance, step class, kickboxing class, boxing class, or any other type of activity that will keep your heart rate elevated at an intermediate-to-high intensity for at least 30 minutes.

The most important thing about planning your weekly exercise program is to make sure that it fits into your life, and that it's structured in a way that suits you best, so you will be sure to stick to it.

4. Nutrition: You Are What You Eat

Aside from taking the time once a week to plan and shop for healthy meals for the week ahead, the single best thing you can do for your diet is to stay aware of the foods you're putting into your body. You learned a lot over the course of my program, and it's important to remember the basics as you move forward:

- Be mindful when you eat so you make the right choices. This is not the time to stuff your face with the first thing you get your hands on. Think before you eat. Think about your goals, your health, your future, your family, and your body.
- Read labels and ingredients lists carefully and choose foods wisely. If you know that an ingredient does not occur in nature—or you just can't pronounce it—chances are you do not want to put it into your body.
- Reduce the amount of toxins and harmful chemicals that make their way into your body by choosing unprocessed and organic food whenever you can.
- Consume the right amount—and the right kinds—of protein, fats, and carbs so that you are getting your healthy nutrients in the correct and balanced proportions. Review Part 3 for exact proportions.
- Consume 25 to 32 grams of fiber a day (for women), and 45 grams per day (for men).
- Hydrate, hydrate, hydrate! Drink half of your body weight in ounces of water daily.

- Take a multivitamin every day.
- Reduce your sugar intake to 15 grams or less per serving of food.
- Limit your intake of alcohol to one or two servings a week. Better yet, eliminate alcohol altogether.
- Increase meal frequency as you decrease portion size. Remember, you don't have to eat until you are full, just until you are satisfied. Only eat half of your plate when you are dining out. Eat five or six smaller meals a day rather than two or three big ones to help accelerate your metabolism and keep your body burning those calories.

Perhaps the most important things to remember when it comes to your diet are portion control, moderation, and quality wholesome food. The food you eat every day affects your immediate and long-term health, and if you abuse your body now, you will have to pay later.

5. COMMIT AND BE CONSISTENT

Nothing will work unless you do.

—*Maya Angelou*

Now that you've completed the life-changing twenty-one-day program, it's especially important to remember the commitment you've made to get yourself to this point, and to remain consistent about doing what needs to be done to honor that commitment. Take time to schedule your workouts. Your workouts are just as important as anything else in your calendar, so don't skip them and don't pass them up for other appointments or meetings. Plan and shop for meals for the week ahead. You'll be amazed at how much a little forward thinking can do when it comes to your kitchen and your diet. Remember, if you take the time to look after yourself first, you will be a better person for everyone else in your life.

It's also important to remember that one bad day, or even one bad week, is *not the end of the world,* nor is it the end of your lifelong journey toward mental and physical health and wellness. After all, you are only human. If you stray from your new healthy habits, don't despair and give up. If you stay committed to changing your schedule and your lifestyle, eating well and exercising will eventually become a part of your life, like taking a shower or brushing your teeth. Remember the Aristotle quote that started this whole journey: "We are what we repeatedly do. Excellence, therefore, is not an act, but a habit." If you stay committed and consistent, your life *will* keep changing for the better.

6. EDUCATE YOURSELF

A book tightly shut is but a block of paper.

—*Chinese proverb*

Research about health and fitness is constantly expanding what we know about how to take care of ourselves. So you need to take responsibility for your health and your life by seeking out the most credible information from reliable sources. Keep up an open dialogue with your doctor or health-care professional, and ask lots of questions. Don't let anyone take away your power to choose what you put into your body, whether it's food or pharmaceuticals. Knowledge is power!

I recommend the following books, audio CDs, and Web sites as sources of helpful, accessible, and reliable information:

BOOKS AND AUDIO CDS

Antioxidants: The Real Story by Michael Colgan, M.D., Apple Publishing, 1999.

Beat Arthritis by Michael Colgan, M.D., Apple Publishing, 1999.

The Cholesterol Myths: Exposing the Fallacy that Saturated Fat and Cholesterol Cause Heart Disease by Uffe Ravnskov, M.D., Ph.D., New Trends Publishing, Inc., 2000.

The Complete Book of Food Counts, 7th Edition by Corrine T. Netzer, Dell, 2005.

Creating Affluence: The A-to-Z Steps to a Richer Life by Deepak Chopra, New World Library and Amber-Allen Publishing, 1998.

Dr. Andrew Weil's Guide to Optimum Health: A Complete Course on How to Feel Better, Live Longer, and Enhance Your Health Naturally (unabridged audio) by Andrew Weil, M.D., Sounds True, 2002.

Dr. Mercola's Total Health Program by Joseph Mercola, M.D., et al. Mercola.com, 2003.

Fats That Heal and Fats That Kill by Udo Erasmus, M.D., Burnaby, Alive Books, 1993.

The Four Agreements: A Practical Guide to Personal Freedom (A Toltec Wisdom Book) by Don Miguel Ruiz, Amber-Allen Publishing, 1997.

Healthy Aging: A Lifelong Guide to Your Physical and Spiritual Well-Being by Andrew Weil, M.D., Alfred A. Knopf, 2005.

Heart Disease by Uffe Ravnskov, M.D., Ph.D., New Trends Publishing, Inc., 2000.

Hormonal Health by Michael Colgan, M.D., Apple Publishing, 1996.

How to Eat, Move and Be Healthy! by Paul Chek, C.H.E.K. Institute, 2004.

Know Your Fats: The Complete Primer for Understanding the Nutrition of Fats, Oils, and Cholesterol by Mary G. Enig, Ph.D., Bethesda Press, 2004.

The Metabolic Typing Diet by Trish Fahey and William Linz Wolcott, Doubleday, 2000.

Nutrition and Physical Degeneration by Weston A. Price, M.D., Price-Pottenger Nutrition Foundation, 1981.

Protect Your Prostate by Michael Colgan, M.D., Apple Publishing, 2000.

The Purpose Driven Life: What on Earth Am I Here For? Rick Warren, Zondervan, 2002.

The Right Protein by Michael Colgan, M.D., Apple Publishing, 1999.

The Seat of the Soul by Gary Zukav, Simon & Schuster, 1999.

The Seven Spiritual Laws of Success: A Practical Guide to the Fulfillment of Your Dreams (based on Creating Affluence) by Deepak Chopra, Amber-Allen Publishing, 1998.

Sports Nutrition Guide by Michael Colgan, M.D., Apple Publishing, 2002.

SuperFoods Rx: Fourteen Foods That Will Change Your Life by Steven Pratt, M.D., and Kathy Matthews, William Morrow, 2003.

The 24-Hour Turnaround: The Formula for Permanent Weight Loss, Antiaging and Optimal Health—Starting Today by Jay Williams, Ph.D., Regan Books, 2002.

The Untold Story of Milk: Green Pastures, Contented Cows and Raw Dairy Products by Ron Schmid, N.D., New Trends Publishing, Inc., 2003.

Water and Salt: The Essence of Life by Peter Ferreira and Barbara Hendel, Natural Resources, 2003.

The Wisdom of Menopause: Creating Physical and Emotional Health and Healing During the Change by Christiane Northrup, M.D., Bantam, 2006.

You Are What You Eat (audio CD) by Paul Chek available at www.chekinstitute.com

Your Body's Many Cries for Water by Fereydoon Batmanghelidj, M.D., Global Health Solutions, 1995.

WEB SITES

www.thehollywoodtrainer.com: the Web site for Jeanette Jenkins and The Hollywood Trainer™

www.ahealthybet.com: BET Foundation's A Healthy BET is a national campaign devoted to promoting healthy eating and lifestyle habits to reduce the occurrences of obesity among African-Americans. The program includes celebrity and real-life public service and programming vignettes on the BET network, a nationwide fitness challenge, community forums on nutrition and fitness, a journal/brochure, and a toll-free information line, as well as the dedicated Web site, which offers health information, videos, and articles.

www.bet.com: the Health channel located on this Web site for BET television, featuring a range of health information along with the BET Foundation's A Healthy BET

www.newleaffitness.com: the official Web site of New Leaf Fitness, which provides education and locations for active (cardiorespiratory test) and resting metabolic tests

www.calorieking.com or www.fitday.com: provides online calorie counters

www.price-pottenger.org: the Price-Pottenger Nutrition Foundation site and online bookstore

www.realmilk.com: the Real Milk campaign promoting humane, nontoxic, pasture-based dairying and small-scale traditional processing

www.colganinstitute.com: Dr. Michael Colgan, author

www.watercure.com: Dr. Fereydoon Batmanghelidj, author

www.humankinetics.com: online bookstore, seminars, and health education networks

www.ideafit.com: the Web site of IDEA, the world's largest association for health and fitness professionals, which publishes journals, hosts fitness conventions, and provides sources for fitness trainers and other fitness news and information

www.ecaworldfitness.com: the Web site of East Coast Alliance World Fitness Association, which conducts conferences, workshops, and conventions to provide education for the fitness industry

www.mercola.com: Dr. Joseph Mercola's newsletter and Web site, which is dedicated to guiding consumers to achieve a high level of health and wellness without expensive drugs or surgery

www.cdc.gov: the Centers for Disease Control

www.webMD.com: one of the largest Web sites providing a wide range of general medical information

www.drlenkravitz.com: Dr. Len Kravitz, author and educator, provides health and fitness education to exercise enthusiasts, fitness instructors, and personal trainers. In this site you will find questions and answers, selected articles by Dr. Kravitz, an online health resource library, and some fitness, health, and exercise physiology trivia tests.

www.ihpfit.com: the Web site of Juan Carlos Santana and the Institute of Human Performance, which is a leading Functional Training facility, providing seminars, workshops, and DVDs

www.nasm.com: National Academy of Sports Medicine

www.acsm.org: American Council of Sports Medicine

www.afaa.com: Aerobics and Fitness Association of America

www.cooperinst.org: the Cooper Institute in Dallas, Texas, founded by Dr. Kenneth Cooper, is dedicated to advancing the understanding of the relationship between living habits and health and to providing leadership in implementing these concepts to enhance the physical and emotional well-being of individuals.

www.mayoclinic.com: the Web site of the Mayo Clinic, the not-for-profit medical center dedicated to the diagnosis and treatment of virtually every type of complex illness, providing tools to consumers for healthier lives

www.stottpilates.com: Stott Pilates equipment, DVDs, and educational seminars

www.performbetter.com: books, equipment, DVDs, and educational seminars

www.collage.com: Collage Videos, featuring an extensive collection of exercise DVDs

7. CREATE A SUPPORTIVE ENVIRONMENT

The seventh point of the star reminds us to build a supportive, loving, positive environment in which your new self can flourish. Continue to reach out and extend the network of people who can help and inspire you as you move forward on the journey you have just begun. You've succeeded so far—having people around you to encourage you and keep you on track will help ensure that you keep succeeding for the rest of your long, healthy, and happy life.

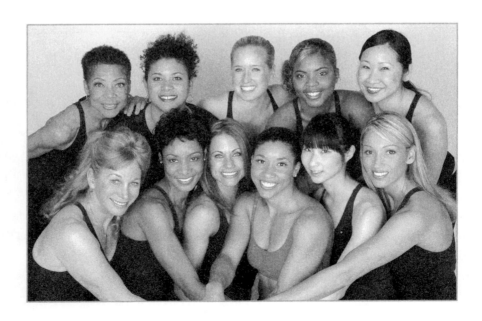

APPENDIX: THE FORMS

Use the following forms to track your progress. You can photocopy the forms or download them from www.thehollywoodtrainer.com.

FORM 7: DAILY FOOD LOG

The following chart should be used to record breakfast, lunch, dinner, and snacks, as well as the nutritional content and value of each food you eat. This form can be photocopied or downloaded from www.thehollywoodtrainer.com.

Every day, you will want to keep the following questions in mind. The more mindful you are of your food intake, the more successful you will be.

How many times did I eat today?

Did I eat within my daily calorie allotment? If not, what could I have done to decrease the amount of calories I consumed?

Did I consume any food item(s) that contained omega-3 essential fatty acids?

How many grams of fiber and how many grams of sugar did I consume today?

Did I eat my daily recommended amount of protein based on my ideal weight?

How many fresh fruits and vegetables did I eat today?

What are some changes, if any, I can make to improve the quality of food that I eat today?

Date:

Total Daily Food Calories you can consume from your Calorie Intake and Output Chart (Form 5):

Goal Water Intake:

Actual Water Intake:

	Food	Time
BREAKFAST		
SNACK		
LUNCH		
SNACK		
SNACK		
DINNER		

Food Items	CALORIES	PROTEIN	CARBOHYDRATES	FIBER	SUGAR	FAT	SODIUM	PROCESSED OR WHOLE FOOD	CONVENTIONAL OR ORGANIC
Total									

FORM 8: CARDIORESPIRATORY TRAINING LOG—CARDIO BURN WORKOUT

Use the following chart to record your workouts. This form can be photocopied or downloaded from www.thehollywoodtrainer.com.

Your Initial VO2max score and rating:

Your Heart Rate Training Zones

Aerobic Base Training Zone 50–75% Heart Rate Max:

Intermediate-to-Advanced Aerobic Training Zone 65–85% Heart Rate Max:

Interval Training Zone 70–90% Heart Rate Max:

DATE											
WORKOUT TIME											
LENGTH OF WORKOUT											
CARDIO BURN WORKOUT LEVEL											
HEART RATE AT 5 MINUTES											
AT 10 MINUTES											
AT 20 MINUTES											
AT 25 MINUTES											
1 MINUTE AFTER WORKOUT (COOLDOWN)											
2 MINUTES AFTER WORKOUT (COOLDOWN)											
3 MINUTES AFTER WORKOUT (COOLDOWN)											

FORM 9: CIRCUIT TRAINING LOG

Use the following charts to record your workouts. This form can be photocopied or downloaded from www.thehollywoodtrainer.com. Take your time to execute each exercise with good form and technique.

Keep the following question in mind to ensure that you are achieving maximum results:

Did I feel challenged?

To increase challenge, you can:

1. Increase the number of reps.
2. Increase the weight.
3. Move quickly from one exercise to the next without taking a break.
4. Focus on your form and make sure you are recruiting the right muscles to execute the movement.

Notes:

CHEST, TRI'S, AND BOOTY CIRCUIT

Date:

Circuit Level (1–5):

Start Time:

	1st Set		2nd Set		1st Set		2nd Set	
	WEIGHT	REPS	WEIGHT	REPS	WEIGHT	REPS	WEIGHT	REPS
PUSH-UP (MODIFIED OR FULL)								
BACK KICKS								
CRUNCHES								
CHEST FLYS								
REVERSE LUNGES								
REPEATER KNEES	CARDIO							
OVERHEAD PRESSES								
SQUATS								
ALTERNATING KNEE-UPS	CARDIO							
OVERHEAD TRICEPS EXTENSIONS								
SINGLE LEG REACHES								
STANDING OBLIQUE CRUNCHES	CARDIO							
TRICEPS KICKBACKS								
SINGLE LEG SQUATS								
CROSS TORSO REPEATER KNEE	CARDIO							
TIME TO COMPLETE SET								
DID YOU DO ANY DROP SETS?								

Time to complete both sets:

BACK, BI'S, AND THIGHS CIRCUIT

Date:

Circuit Level (1–5):

Start Time:

	1st Set		2nd Set		1st Set		2nd Set	
	WEIGHT	REPS	WEIGHT	REPS	WEIGHT	REPS	WEIGHT	REPS
BACK FLYS								
PLIÉ SQUATS								
ALTERNATING KNEE-UPS	CARDIO							
BACK ROWS								
STATIONARY LUNGES								
LATERAL SIDE SHUFFLES	CARDIO							
UPRIGHT ROWS								
OUTER THIGH LEG LIFTS								
TOUCH HEEL REPEATER KNEES	CARDIO							
BICEP CURLS								
INNER THIGH								
STANDING OBLIQUE CRUNCHES	CARDIO							
EXTERNAL ROTATION AND REACH (SHOULDERS AND BACK)								
CROSS TORSO REPEATER KNEES	CARDIO							
LEG SCISSORS	NO WEIGHT							
TIME TO COMPLETE SET								
DID YOU DO ANY DROP SETS?								

Time to complete both sets:

FORM 10: FLEXIBILITY TRAINING LOG

Use the following chart to record your workouts. This form can be photocopied or downloaded from www.thehollywoodtrainer.com. Take your time to execute each stretch with good form and technique.

Keep the following questions in mind to ensure that you are achieving maximum results:

What areas do I feel need additional stretching?

Are there any areas that were not stretched in which I felt pain or stiffness?

Notes about areas that I would like to put more focus on:

Date	LENGTH OF TIME HOLDING STRETCH											
Straddle Stretch Center												
Straddle Stretch Right												
Straddle Stretch Left												
Forward Flexion, Right Knee Bent												
Forward Flexion, Flexion, Left Knee Bent												
Right Quadriceps Stretch												
Left Quadriceps Stretch												
Cross-Legged Stretch, Right Leg												

Date												
Cross-Legged Stretch, Left Leg												
Right Hamstring Stretch												
Left Hamstring Stretch												
Right Buttocks Stretch												
Left Buttocks Stretch												
Spinal Rotation, Right Side												
Spinal Rotation, Left Side												
Cobra Stretch (Abs)												
Cat Stretch (Lower Back)												
Right Calf Stretch												
Left Calf Stretch												
Chest and Front Deltoid right												
Chest and Front Deltoid left												
Bicep and Forearm right												
Bicep and Forearm left												

Date											
Right Triceps											
Left Triceps											
Upper Back											
Right Rear Deltoid and Triceps											
Left Rear Deltoid and Triceps											
Right Neck Stretches											
Left Neck Stretches											

FORM 11: BEFORE-AND-AFTER PHOTOS

Watch your body change as you change your life. Make seven photocopies of this form. Take four photos of yourself—front view, left side view, right side view, and back view—and paste them in the appropriate boxes. Make sure that you are wearing a bathing suit, bikini, or formfitting workout bra and shorts. (If you cover yourself up it will be more difficult to see the physical changes in your body; these are the changes that you will not see on the scale, but you will be amazed when you look back at your photos.) Photocopy this form and put it into the Measurements section of your journal, along with new photos you take every six weeks. Mark your calendar so you don't forget.

Photo 1: Front View   *Photo 2: Back View*

Photo 3: Right Side View   *Photo 4: Left Side View*

ACKNOWLEDGMENTS

I would like to thank:

God for using me to motivate others to live healthy lifestyles and for the opportunity to get back up with hope every time I fall!

My family, who has taught me how to love: my mom, Karen Jones, my brother, Roger Jenkins, and my sister, Camille Watson.

My college buddy and business partner, Melinda Travis, and her husband, Curtis Travis, who have always believed in and supported my dreams.

Queen Latifah, Shakim Compere, Mrs. Owens, and the Team 'tifah family and crew for opening their hearts and treating me as a member of the family.

My angel investors and clients who supported me in my first project: Dana Owens, Magic Johnson, Terrell Owens, Taryn Manning, Amy Weber, Rayetta Seals, Kristy Lees, Alan Watson, Dominique Appleby, Gayle Heaney, Amy Plummer, Traci Mendez, John Busigin, Ralph Cuglietta, Petri Lasi, Eric Wycoff, Helga Magliolo, Marcel Patterson, Kimber Lee Renay Floyd, Helene Rosenzweig, Sal Tuzzolino, the Silberman family, the Essakow family, and the Helfet family.

My awesome executive assistants, Carla Kemp, Monica Keller Rodriguez, Brely Evans, and Erin Tompkins.

My managers at Associated Talent Management.

My publisher, John Duff, for his dedication and constructive feedback.

All of my students, clients, and friends who have permitted me to share their amazing stories: Angela Magliocco, Brely Evans, Amber Dykes, Myron Harris, Liz Scott, Marsha Fiacconi, Taji Tortorello, Kim Lohrke, Barbara Bagneris, Charley Johnson, Heather Funston, Noemy, and Tanya.

BET, BET Foundation, and BET.com for allowing me the opportunity to give the gift of health and fitness to the African American community through your various media outlets. Debra Lee, Stephen Hill, Reginald Hudlin, Kelli Lawson, Rodney Gill, Sonia Lockett, Lynda Dorman, Vicki Johnson, Lyntina Townsend, and One 9.

Lifetime Television for the opportunity to host the new and exciting exercise program.

National Urban League, Urban Influence Magazine, and Tamara Brown.

Michelle McIvor and the staff of iVillage.com.

Doug Smith and the staff of Lady Foot Locker.

Lori Roth and the staff of Nike for supporting me in my crazy projects over the years; you guys are the best!

Pietown Productions and the Food Network for offering me the opportunity to be a part of "Weighing In."

The staff of New Leaf Fitness: Rod Young, Terry Kapsen, Tim Quinn, Sean Sutter, and Gary McCoy, for your support in all of my many projects as we continue to educate and motivate people to learn about their metabolic rates.

All of the television producers, editors, writers, radio hosts, and producers who have profiled my work over the years.

My backup talent and friends Cheyenne Kidd, Richard Lee Aaron Curtis IV, Charley Johnson, Tanja Djelevic, Kimberly Floyd, Babatunde Oyedokum, Erin Omar, Brely Evans, Nathalie Ames, Angel Ramos, and Alex Couchonnal.

Mike Leber and Stock Yard Films for your great work in producing the DVD that goes with this book and for putting up with my crazy schedule.

Musicflex Music.

Jeff Hays, Alan Winters, Teri Sundh, and the staff and owners of Pod Fitness for your support, energy, drive, and positive outlook!

June Evans and Kim Young for allowing me the opportunity to get involved with the "Love My Body" Campaign!

Sharon House and the staff of Much and House Public Relations for supporting me and the Hollywood Trainer company over the years.

The staff and owners of Crunch, the Fitness Factory, and Sports Club LA for allowing me the opportunity to jump around in Lycra all day and inspire people to live healthy lifestyles!

My agent, Andy Barvzi—and Harley Pasternak for making the connection.

My colleagues. You have all inspired me in so many ways. Keep doing your thing! Kendell Hogan, Donna Cyrus, Pat Soley, Michelle Lemay, Patrick Goudeau, Calvin Wiley, Karen Voight, Phillip Gray, Billy Blanks and staff, Greg Isaac, Jay Blahnik, Juliane Arney, Petra Kolber, Lisa Wheeler, Michael George, Kathy Smith, Dr. Ro, Dr. Jay Williams, Rob Glick, Harley Pasternak, Gunnar Peterson, Donna Richardson, Madonna Grimes, Mocha Lee, Yumi Lee, Ron Matthews, Linda Shelton, Douglas Brooks, Todd Durkin, Nancy Kennedy, Bobby Storm, Ashley Borden, BJ Burns, Keli Roberts, Lawrence Biscontini, Steven Earth, Darin Chandler, Andrea Orbeck, Kristy Lees, Bob Harper, John Garey, and many more, I am sure!

All my teachers, educators, and coaches at G. L. Roberts High School in Oshawa, Ontario; Ridgemont High School in Ottawa, Ontario; the University of Ottawa; and UCLA; as well as those who continue to educate me today: Dr. Joseph Mercola, Paul Chek, Dr. Walter Willet, Dr. Len Kravitz, Beth Shaw and the Yogafit program, Moira Stott and the Stott Pilates program, Dr. Weston Price and the Price-Pottenger Foundation, Dr. Reed, Joshua Rosenthal and the School of Integrative Nutrition, Dr. James Walton, Deepak Chopra, Oprah Winfrey, Dr. Andrew Weil, Dr. Christiane Northrup, Dr. Fereydoon Batmanghelidj, Dr. Steven Pratt, William Wolcott, and Dr. Roger Williams.

The staff of IDEA Health and Fitness and ECA (East Coast Alliance).

INDEX

RECIPES INDEX

ABOUT THE AUTHOR

Jeanette Jenkins, founder and president of The Hollywood Trainer™, is the host of Lifetime Television's *My Workout: Powered by Podfitness* and fitness coach for the ivillage.com *iLose It for Good* Community Challenge®. Jenkins is a Nike Elite Athlete, a Podfitness.com premier trainer, and the official spokesperson for the BET Foundation's A Healthy BET campaign. Her expertise as a fitness and nutritional consultant has been featured on *The Tonight Show with Jay Leno, Extra, Access Hollywood,* and *The Tyra Banks Show;* Food Network, VH1, and BET; and Oprah.com, MSNBC.com, eDiets.com, and ivillage.com. Her work has been profiled in *O, The Oprah Magazine, InStyle, Fitness, Shape, Self, Redbook, Glamour, Cosmopolitan Style & Beauty, Essence,* and other publications. She writes regular columns for the Los Angeles *Daily News, Urban Influence, Precious Times,* and MSNBC.com, among others. Jenkins, who has worked with Queen Latifah, actress Taryn Manning, swimsuit model Amy Weber, several NFL and NBA athletes, and many other celebrities, studied human kinetics at the University of Ottawa and holds more than seventeen international certifications in nutrition and various fitness training methods. She lives in Los Angeles.

Visit the author's website at www.thehollywoodtrainer.com.